The Art of
Spiritual Midwifery

The Art of
Spiritual Midwifery

diaLogos and Dialectic in the Classical Tradition

Stephen Faller

CASCADE Books • Eugene, Oregon

THE ART OF SPIRITUAL MIDWIFERY
diaLogos and Dialectic in the Classical Tradition

Copyright © 2015 Stephen Faller. All rights reserved. Except for brief quotations in critical publications or reviews, no part of this book may be reproduced in any manner without prior written permission from the publisher. Write: Permissions, Wipf and Stock Publishers, 199 W. 8th Ave., Suite 3, Eugene, OR 97401.

Cascade Books
An Imprint of Wipf and Stock Publishers
199 W. 8th Ave., Suite 3
Eugene, OR 97401

www.wipfandstock.com

ISBN 13: 978-1-62564-887-7

Cataloguing-in-Publication data:

Faller, Stephen.

    The art of spiritual midwifery : diaLogos and dialectic in the classical tradition / Stephen Faller.

    xvi + 254 pp. ; 23 cm. Includes bibliographical references.

    ISBN 13: 978-1-62564-887-7

    1. Spiritual direction. 2. Midwifery—Spiritual aspects. 3. Jesus Christ. 4. Socrates. I. Title.

BV5053 .F37 2015

Manufactured in the U.S.A.

For Heather.

Socrates: How absurd of you, never to have heard that I am the son of a midwife, a fine buxom woman called Phaenarete!

Theaetetus: I have heard that.

Socrates: Have you also been told that I practice the same art?

Theaetetus: No, never.

Socrates: It is true, though; only don't give away my secret. It is not known that I possess this skill; so the ignorant world describes me in other terms as an eccentric person who reduces people to hopeless perplexity. Have you been told that too?

Theaetetus: I have.

Socrates: Consider, then, how it is with all midwives; that will help you to understand what I mean. I dare say you know that they never attend other women in childbirth so long as they themselves can conceive and bear children, but only when they are too old for that . . . . My art of midwifery is in general like theirs; the only difference is that my patients are men, not women, and my concern is not with the body but with the soul that is in the travail of birth . . . . I am so far like the midwife that I myself cannot give birth to wisdom, and the common reproach is true, that though I question others, I can myself bring nothing to light because there is no wisdom in me.

    The reason is this. Heaven constrains me to serve as a midwife, but has debarred me from giving birth. So of myself I have no sort of wisdom, nor has any discovery ever been born to me as the child of my soul. Those who frequent my company at first appear, some of them, quite unintelligent, but, as we go further with our discussions, all who are favored by heaven make progress at a rate that seems surprising to others as well as to themselves, although it is clear that they have never learned anything from me. The many admirable truths they bring to birth have been discovered by themselves from within. But the delivery is heaven's work and mine.

Contents

Attunement | ix

Part I: Poetics, Aesthetics, and Ethics | 1
   1 The Midwife | 3
   2 The Baby | 12
   3 Medicine and Dialogue | 22

Part II: Physique and Physics | 39
   4 The How and the What | 41
   5 The Pangs of Socratic Irony | 49
   6 Seduction, Surrender, and Negation | 62
   7 Inductive Logic and Being Induced | 73

Part III: Immanence and Emanations | 83
   8 Lighting and Dark Sayings | 85
   9 The Center | 96
  10 Precepts, Forceps, and Applications | 102

     Afterward and Afterword: The Symposium | 113
     Bibliography | 141

Attunement

> Men do not know how
> what is at variance
> agrees with itself.
> It is an attunement of opposite tension,
> like that of the bow and the lyre.
>
> HERACLITUS

THE TUNING OF AN orchestra is a more recognizable performance than any familiar symphony to follow. It is unmistakable; yet there is no score. Each tune up is different, and those in the audience can tease out the different instruments—all those sounds are there for the sifting. Noise gives way to the discovery of notes. And yet wherever this happens anywhere in the world, it is obvious what is going on.

Perhaps we can explain this phenomenon by saying that if you were to hear this once, forever would you know that there is only one possible explanation for that kind of noise and cacophony. We can say that the noise is so bad that it is forever seared into the mind and for that reason it strikes us as unforgettable and unmistakable.

But this traumatic disclaimer fails to resonate with our highest intimation and the deeper intuition. Simply, a tuning orchestra doesn't sound that bad. It sounds kind of fun and playful. It conveys an almost spiritual striving for an ideal as the strings are tightened, and as the keys are turned a keen listening is happening.

No. Not quite. A little more. There.

Attunement

Perhaps what is most recognizable is the human struggle for attunement. The search for balance. This inquiry into spiritual midwifery in the classical tradition relies on that kind of balance and tension.

Form and Function

Theological books have changed. While we may go through tomes of systematic theology as part of the graduate level education (although it is more likely that we go through chosen excerpts), the kind of text that today's practical theologian reaches for as a field guide has changed considerably. Gone are the pages and pages of abstract theology that might be found in Tillich. There is no longer the comprehensiveness of Calvin or Barth. We no longer wade through the Victorian prose of Wesley. And Kierkegaard's idea of spiritual formation and training through a readership would never work today. The written word has changed. It looks different. It's organized differently. Its function is different. It's written for the reader who is "on the go." There are subheads and subdivisions, all structured to help the reader find something quickly—and it better be useful.

Herein lies a peculiar tension. Because anyone who is any good at this curious work of the care of souls knows that quick answers don't work—and that has probably been true since the book of Job. Any therapeutic or transformative process is actually hindered and encumbered by the easy answer. These simple ideas of the obvious create resentment, resistance, and spiritual blockages for all those who must endure them. These quick answers short circuit the labyrinth-like journey on which the soul must go.

So here's the question: if we know that easy answers don't work when we are offering pastoral care or in doing some type of counseling, why does today's literature gravitate toward that kind of writing? How can authors say all there is to say but expect their readers to not say too much? Most texts today have a little bit of telling theory with some intricacy, but instead of taking the reader on a journey they put in just enough case studies so that the theory feels like a narrative.

As we go forward, this will be one of the central tensions that we hold. This is meant to be an applied resource and it therefore must be accessible and comprehensible. But at the same time, there is an implicit understanding that the subject matter is numinous and large. There must be a little bit of mystery in a manual about the care of souls. And to preserve that mystery, we're going to look for tensile language and multivalent metaphor.

Attunement

In a beginner's creative writing class, the constant admonition is "Show, don't tell." We live in an instant coffee kind of culture, where everything is on demand, and we expect to be told, and hunger for the tell-all. This is where we are. So you can expect both show and tell.

More pointedly, there are some tensions here that I want you to hold with me. My project does build an argument, but I am asking you to circumambulate with me along a discursive path. I'm introducing a significant concept, but feel the need to preserve digressive movements that are a natural part of any dialogue. I'm charged with the task of providing credible information, but I'm asking to offer the gift of formation.

Midwifery and Pastoral Care

One of the things that became apparent in this study is that the intrinsic metaphor here, that of the midwife, is problematic. This is the metaphor before us today, this is the metaphor that we receive from Jesus and Socrates.

Here's why the metaphor is problematic: a metaphor rightly consists of a vehicle and a tenor—that is, a meaning. Midwifery is our vehicle, and its implied context of birth easily overpowers its tenor, which seems to be an abstract technique in the care of souls. Birth is an existential and experiential reality with powerful memories engrafted into our very bodies.

Simply put, you can have a book about midwifery, even spiritual midwifery, without ever referencing Jesus or Socrates. And those books and articles have been written in the spiritual direction literature by Margaret Guenther, Karen Hanson, and others. But the converse is not true; you cannot have a book about this Socratic approach without returning to the vitality of the metaphor. Socrates needs the metaphor in a way that the metaphor does not need Socrates. There are specific ideas, structures, and techniques mapped out by Socrates but they are all enhanced by a rich appreciation of the metaphor. Sometimes it is not yet clear how the theories apply and the only guide we have is the metaphor of the midwife.

In the *Phaedrus*, Socrates says the following about metaphor: "To tell what it really is would be a theme for a divine and a very long discourse; what it resembles, however, may be expressed more briefly and in human language."[1] He's saying that we are constrained to the world of metaphor. We have to find comparisons.

---

1. Plato, *Phaedrus*, 28.

Attunement

This is not a book that seeks to tell the truth about women's bodies. That is a profound truth, resting quietly beyond the capability of this author. But that said, the collective influence of the Jesus movement and the Socrates movement has been enormous. If for no other reason than the caliber of who is speaking, an audience is demanded. This is a tenor that is powerful and can be amplified within this metaphor. Simply, they are describing a profound subject, which will be our subject if possible, and the metaphor for this is midwifery.

It is also worth noting, repeatedly, that Jesus and Socrates were men. Midwifery typically belongs to women. What's going on here? There is a problem here, but the problem is not an accident of the work. It is the work.

It's also probably true that women who are spiritual caregivers have also embraced midwifery as a metaphor for many of the same reasons. Some readers remind me of the neglected nature of women's work. The neglect is real, metaphorically and otherwise. Many spiritual directors are a part of theological traditions that question the spiritual authority of women, and so spiritual midwifery remains as an understated power.

If we wanted to be gender accurate, we could constrain spiritual midwifery to women and something else to men. Fatherhood is not the right relation; that analog goes with motherhood. But we could come up with some kind of husbandry if we needed to say that there was a spiritual work that typically fell to men.

But it remains very significant that neither Jesus nor Socrates took that recourse. They, very much as men, wanted this feminine metaphor, this rhetorical gender-bending. Those who heard their language were confounded, and it seems as though not accidently. Margaret Guenther, who has done groundbreaking work in spiritual direction, also has explored the treasures of the midwifery metaphor. She says, "Like the midwife, spiritual directors are with-women and with-men. While biological birthgiving is the prerogative of the female and midwives are traditionally female, in the ministry of spiritual direction, anatomy is not destiny."[2] It is my hope, as a male author, that she is right, and that these luminaries that I so admire, like Jesus and Socrates, can be held creatively with this metaphor that I respect and this image that humbles me.

And while this is not a book that can tell the truth about women's bodies, this is a book about spiritual midwifery, and this historical nugget in the tradition of the care of souls so readily benefits from its conjoined

2. Guenther, *Holy Listening*, loc. 1040–41.

connection to the metaphor. Time and again, the comparison to the art of the midwife shows a new insight and manifests a different value that is congruent with the methodology we are exploring. Indeed, much about midwifery is a lost art. For centuries, women have carried this information from one generation to the next, whispered over cries, transmitted during transition, and told as contractions take hold. That information and wisdom is largely lost to us today. We don't see much about birth in popular culture; birth seems anything but natural.

And spiritual midwifery also conveys a wisdom that has been lost, but it has certainly been out there for all to see since the beginnings of Western civilization. The texts are there and have been there. But other questions have taken center stage and spiritual midwifery has become hidden, buried, and forgotten—certainly only more so in the last hundred years.

And the point is that this is another rich point of comparison between this vehicle and this tenor that add to the power of this metaphor. And there are many more comparisons. So in many ways, this book about the care of souls so very much is and is not about midwifery.

History and Practice

As my research unfolded, so did my excitement about this unappreciated gem in the history of pastoral care. My research became influenced by all kinds of projections I had toward my subject. I began to see it as a maligned orphan, an idea birthed by the worthiest of worthies only to be abandoned to historical obscurity. But when you allow those projections to take hold, you can't describe your research effectively and you sound like a wild-eyed conspiracy theorist.

Reviewing the historical development of an idea is not necessarily the best way to communicate either the idea itself or its useful demonstration. In other words, getting wrapped up in the need to establish a historical foundation for spiritual midwifery is essentially a different project than creating a tool to teach it. That project has an academic quality and academic motivations that really don't fit here. There are also academic maneuvers, to which we are not confined. We are not required to find consensus, nor constrained to certainty. Indeed, the academic argument is something that can be fought and won, but spiritual midwifery isn't about winning.

But it is neither the case that the historical context is irrelevant, nor that it is unimportant. The historical context can clarify the ideas and contextualize what is being said. The historical context can elucidate the theory, and it's the theory that forms the practice. Again, you can be so theoretical as to cloud and confuse the practice, but you do need some kind of theoretical frame of sufficient rigor that can help you inhabit the practice. As the practice gets into difficulty you need a strong enough theory to guide you through the questions. Theory is important, but the care of souls is not theoretical.

Moreover, the historical story behind spiritual midwifery is itself a story worth telling. It is no small thing that spiritual midwifery attaches itself to such luminaries as Jesus and Socrates. Clearly these figures have made an indelible footprint on the path of Western civilization. It seems to me that anyone in the work would be interested to know more about spiritual midwifery just from its historical import alone.

To be clear: we will not be exploring the history of everything that has ever been called spiritual midwifery. There are specific ideas, concepts, technologies and values at the core of the Jesus and Socrates movements, and like the lily to the sun there we turn. When we look at the dialogue and rhetoric accompanying these two traditions, we see both specific instantiation that carries a precise and complex rhetorical technology and a general underlying constellation of values that define a perspective. That's our focus: to look at this kernel coming from the classical tradition because it has been overlooked and hidden. Trying to recover it may even shape living theology today. None of this is meant to marginalize or take away from other excursions into midwifery.

Our project is an applied understanding of spiritual midwifery. There's going to be some history involved. Bringing Heraclitus into the dialogue, for instance, makes the ensuing conversation about midwifery that much richer. And there's going to be some theory because there are some pretty significant ways that the concept of spiritual midwifery runs in a very contrary trajectory to other developments in counseling and the care of souls in the Western tradition.

Religious and Secular

There are always divisions in spirituality and religion. Who is the Christian or pagan? The Jew or Gentile? Where do we draw the line between the sacred and the secular? The *fanum* and the *profanum*?

Attunement

This tension immediately tightens around our discussion of spiritual midwifery. With all of the claims about Jesus that have been made across history, it becomes no small claim to say that this methodology was employed by Jesus. Midwifery is not a Christian commodity, but it ought to be of interest to Christians, especially those who are involved in pastoral care and those who want to offer such care in the name of Christ. And on that point, the obscurity of spiritual midwifery is a most peculiar indictment. If a religion has a founder, and that founder has a demonstrable pattern of working, why has so little attention been paid to that pattern? Nearly half of Jesus' recorded ministry in the Gospels occurs in the same one-on-one paradigm that is so often found in pastoral care. It seems like certain aspects of Jesus' group work, community building, and controversial actions have been highlighted to the exclusion of the lonelier work with individuals. That is most curious.

It is also true that spiritual midwifery in itself does not carry any faith claims about the nature of divinity or the Godhead. To the point, Socrates is able to wield the tool with amazing skill, both as a secular philosopher and as a pious pagan.

It is worth noting that as spiritual midwifery has significant ties to the origins of Western philosophy and Western religion, it is remarkably resonant with religious philosophies in general. Taoism reverberates powerfully with midwifery. The Socratic tradition permeates Islamic philosophy. Dialectical thinking, which lies at the core of spiritual midwifery, has a proud heritage in Buddhist thought. Perhaps the point is as simple as this: the very philosophy and religion embedded in midwifery's history easily engage other sophisticated belief systems, because they are all like parts of like machinery. It translates well because the core technology is native.

It is also important to acknowledge that where matters of Christian interpretation invariably arise because of Jesus' use of spiritual midwifery, those matters will be explored from a Christian perspective. Midwifery inherently calls for integration and embodiment.

But this tension also stretches to the secular. Both Freud and Carl Rogers toyed with the term in describing their work. Who am I to say spiritual midwifery is this and not that?

There are also intrinsic incongruences with the project of academic psychology, not so much because spiritual midwifery is a response to psychology, but because it precedes psychology. Pastoral care and academic psychology have both shared a pragmatic interest in the behavioral sciences, but it may be helpful to remember that these different streams of thought do come from different sources. Some of these incompatibilities will be explored later, but for now it is enough to realize that if the spiritual midwifery directly contrasts to the kind of project of Rogers or Freud, it is needful to realize that we are talking about at least two different things, and fair to wonder who is the rightful holder of the term.

But given the centrality of the Jesus movement and the Socrates movement in the Western tradition, we are justified in saying that there is a definition of spiritual midwifery in the classical tradition, and this is it.

Is and Is Not the Classical Tradition

There remains one more powerful centering paradox as we approach this work. Spiritual midwifery both is and is not a part of the classical Western tradition.

The word *classical* itself is cumbersome because it carries so many superlative associations. The advantage of the word is that it captures the historical period in question. By itself, though, it does not invoke or engage the Jesus tradition. I could have used some Athenian-Judeo construct, but that could have locked the entire conversation into a Judeo-Christian context, and I think the spiritual midwifery is bigger than that. Philosophy and Christianity were later yoked by Rome and centuries of Latin scholarship, although it was Greek that afforded the rhetorical apparatus for the development of Christian theology.

It is not maintained that the "origin" of midwifery is specifically tied to the Jesus or Socrates movement. Both Jesus and Socrates make constant references to sources much older than themselves, and it is tragic that many of those references are lost to us as they are. And this does not seem limited to these thinkers. Lao Tzu frequently refers to the "ancients." These ideas are very, very old, and there are traces of them wherever we find human thought. If religious thought is anchored in mythology, then we can and should dig into the myths behind the myths, out of Rome and into Greece; indeed, out of Greece and into Egypt.

At the same time, something did happen in the course of the Western tradition. If we try to sit back dispassionately and look at the millennia of recorded human history, the intellect initially suggests that human history has unfolded at a uniform rate. Which is fine, except for the fact that that's not how it happened. We know that there are times where not many changes, and then we see periods of tremendous change. Thinkers like Karl Jaspers and Eric Vogelin have coined the terms "Axial Age" and "Great Leap of Being," respectively, to describe the global explosion of philosophy and religion just prior to the classical period. Undeniably, Jesus and Socrates were very important thinkers at a very important time in world history. There is much to be gained from scrutinizing a methodology that they seem to have shared. There are insights to be found of interest to anyone, but also specifically interesting to those who want to make a stand in this tradition particularly—those who celebrate identity here.

But it is hard to make the case that spiritual midwifery is a part of that tradition when it has been traditionally ignored or overlooked. If it is a part of the tradition, it seems to be only in the negative; that spiritual midwifery has been there from the very beginning, and also overlooked from the very beginning.

Many of the academic criticisms of the classical Western tradition (here understood not as the historical events and thinkers themselves, but as the grand Project to assert a conceptual lineage more than a millennium later) may have much light to shed on why midwifery itself has been buried. Insofar as the history of the world is the history of power, it stands to reason that a modality to embrace powerlessness would disappear from the lexicon. If the ideas around the history of power are just as polluted by the power that they are trying to describe, there will be no room for this seeming weakness. The desires of colonial imperialism are essentially incongruent with the accompanying values of spiritual midwifery. Spiritual midwifery is not about taking over the world with an idea.

I'm speaking generally and abstractly here, but this happens in remarkably precise and personal ways. Readers pointed out to me, that if patriarchy has relegated midwifery to "women's work," then that same patriarchy is going to be disinterested in spiritual midwifery; such a patriarchy will have little interest in either the vehicle or the tenor of this metaphor, no matter how beautiful or exquisite either may be.

And this seems exactly right: a negative methodology like midwifery has been there from the beginning.

What's to Come

This work has been divided into three parts. The first part is called, "Poetics, Aesthetics, and Ethics." This metaphor rests in an image, and the image invokes poetics. What is the meaning of the metaphor? Moreover, what does it mean to work with figures of speech like metaphor at all? But if we are dealing with poetics and art and a ministry that claims to be an art, how does the art appear? If the art and art form has a form, how is it, then, that the art is to be formed? And finally, if this complicated art is bound by certain meaning and interpretation, how is it that the art is to be used, both effectively and ethically? If this metaphor offers a prescription, how is the prescription rightly filled?

The second part is called "Physique and Physics." The similarity between the two words already begins to reveal. The essence and science of what something is closely relates to how it moves. The movement shows us anatomy, and anatomy predicts movement. This is the technical part of the work, so there's some theory here. We need to understand as best we can what are the elements of spiritual midwifery, knowing full well that the spirit cannot be placed under a microscope. We need to try to comprehend what the operative forces are, even though the most important forces lie beyond comprehension.

The final part is "Immanence and Emanations." This part is not what the reader may most anticipate: perhaps a comprehensive survey of examples which may illuminate all of the ideas that have been explored. But if this inquiry into spiritual midwifery is only a little accurate; that is, accurate about the human personality and human relationships and human nature, then this endeavor must have all kinds of resonances with the natural world; these emanations must be everywhere. So the third part is more of a springboard than a summary.

Where It Came From

Initial research for this project began in 1999, and the earliest expression of the ideas followed in 2000, although some of the seminal questions can be traced back to 1992. Since these ideas crystallized in 2000, I have had over a decade to experiment, refine, and field test how these concepts really lived, moved, and functioned. I have had the chance to study the pneumakinesthesiology—how the spirit moves and the motion of the soul.

At the beginning, there was a rigid and theoretical quality to the idea of the spiritual midwife—perhaps then as rigid and pristine as one of Plato's forms. And there was a very real disconnect between the abstract idea and the embodied people that I was trying to serve. Over time, and use, things became more ergonomic; the way objects become smooth by wear, like an old, wooden spoon.

A meaningful partnership in this process has always come from the chaplaincy interns that I have worked with since 2002. Since then, some fifty to sixty interns have generously spent their time with me, and several in painstaking detail, trying to flesh out these very ideas. Some of them have labored greatly, to whom I'm greatly indebted.

In trying to explain things, I have been forced to understand myself, again, and again, and again. Sometimes the partnership has worked like polishing sand, and what was needed was a source of friction. Sometimes the partnership has worked by a useful question, a good interrogative light can bring clarity everywhere it shines and especially where it's focused. But in a good number of cases, I learned directly from them, watching them employ the concepts more effectively and adaptively than I ever could have, seeing them achieving transformation in the process of helping others. It is no accident, then, that this resource has evolved as a teaching guide. It is structured to help very busy pastoral caregivers see a very different way of doing pastoral care.

Additionally, this project was significantly enhanced as a granted Pastoral Study Project from the Louisville Institute. Through the grant, there was a Symposium for Spiritual Midwifery, on June 22, 2012. And there are many people to thank for their work at the symposium, which has been partially captured as an afterword to this text.

It might also be helpful to stress that this first volume is only that: a first volume. It is not meant to be exhaustive, and there are many questions that would be missing for it to be so.

The Missing Piece

The dialectical terrain has been initially mapped out, but a piece is missing. From reviewing tomes of husband-coached birthing, one line is seared in my mind: "The prepared husband does not need to ask when sips of water are necessary. That's just sloppy." Much of our preparation deals with the delicate balance of attunement, but the other piece calls for a level of attentiveness that transcends listening. Feel out the needs of this text. Where are its gaps? What is missing? The reader is encouraged and charged to bring that listening to this text, so that the text might become a dialogue. s

Part I
Poetics, Aesthetics, and Ethics

THIS SECTION PLACES CONSIDERABLE emphasis on poetics, aesthetics, and ethics; all three of those play an important role in this first section on spiritual midwifery. I am reminded, for a moment, of Aristotle's categories (he did see fit to address poetics and ethics).

This is a book largely about poetics. Perhaps it's no mistake that Plato had been a poet before he became a disciple of Socrates. I don't think Plato was ever completely able to leave poetry. Much of Platonic philosophy, especially his idea of the forms, is ultimately an assertion of the primacy of poetics. Plato was convinced that our words and ideas pointed to essences that really existed, for example, there was an eternal archetype of a chair, to which all existing chairs somehow conformed. It is a philosophy of meaning and essence. No matter how abstract the idea was, it had a corresponding form, like love or justice. Poetry was powerful because the power was in the words and forms.

There is a primal connection between spirituality and poetry that needs not be forgotten. Whether it's the aboriginal incantation of the shaman or the most abstract doctrine of transubstantiation, both of these belief systems share the core that language has the power over reality.

Poetry itself is a meaningful part of our journey. Poetry and language lie close to the core of our subject. Early on, Jesus and Socrates thought that this kind of work was best named with a metaphor—a figure of speech. Something about this artistic speech is central to the soul work. We are going to have to spend some time understanding figures of speech. Birth is one of the powerful and organic images, period. Indeed, a lot of the

Part I—Poetics, Aesthetics, and Ethics

criticism of my work has stemmed from the sense that it's too powerful of an image for me to wield as a male author. At times, the image seems to overpower the very idea that it's trying to convey. But it should be noted that the spiritual midwifery itself is also extremely powerful.

At the same time, this book is not poetry. Poetry is a certain kind of experience, and this work is not ultimately dedicated to creating that precise experience. That said, this does not mean that there is absolutely no attentiveness to the relationship between form and content or vehicle and tenor. No, this is a book exactly about relationship and especially the in-betweens of relationship. And so, some attention has been dedicated to the matter of aesthetics. Appearances have their place, especially if they succeed in pointing to something beyond appearances.

One disclaimer that fits here is the aesthetic treatment of the dialogical partners. I might quote Socrates, which is really a quote of Plato and the Platonic tradition. I might quote John, and again there is a whole scholastic awareness there. We're not exactly sure that the author of the Gospel of John was the John also mentioned in the Gospels. There's a Johannine tradition there. Okay. But to me, it's John. And Socrates. And Søren. Heraclitus. And Jesus. I don't think I actually achieve anything by reminding readers constantly of the historical uncertainty. Moreover, I have a lot of beliefs about these people. The reader is not expected or required to share those beliefs. Some of the beliefs are historical, some psychological, and some religious. Some of the strongest beliefs are those related to the person of Jesus. Readers might not want to bring a certain analytical perspective to such a religious figure, for a variety of reasons. I certainly mean no disrespect nor slipshod scholarship, but this is exactly how I encounter the historical person of Jesus.

Finally, this is a section that also prescribes its own ethical perspective. There is a way that the midwife works; therefore, there is also a way that the midwife does not work. There is a way that the midwife seeks to facilitate transformation, and there are ways that the midwife is transformed. Focused work asserts responsible work.

Chapter 1

The Midwife

> The mother
> is far enough in front of the child
> so that she cannot actually hold onto the child,
> but she stretches out her arms; she imitates the child's movements.
> If it merely totters,
> she quickly bends as if to grasp it—
> thus the child believes that it is not walking alone.
> The most loving mother can do no more
> if there is to be any truth
> in this matter of the child's walking alone.
>
> KIERKEGAARD

A Brief Description

MY DAUGHTER WAS BORN on Thanksgiving Day, and even though my ministry is hospital based, this was the first birth that I had attended. I suspect everyone remembers the first time they witness a birth. While I had seen videos of birth before, the only way to appreciate the electricity in the room is to be there.

It's difficult to talk about myself. The problem isn't even "oneself"—no, the problem is my self and my particularity. And we'll touch on this several times throughout, but we are dealing with a metaphor that literally drives people to their own experience. I am an author, locked into my experience, seeking to use a metaphor that drives readers to their experience. Hopefully,

Part I—Poetics, Aesthetics, and Ethics

somehow, this can be our metaphor. Spiritual director Margaret Guenther concedes readily, "It is all too easy to see the birth imagery in Scripture (and in the language of popular piety) as abstract, bloodless, remote from human experience. Yet if I were to name my own most profound spiritual or theological experience, without hesitation I would cite the birth of my three children."[1] To be sure, there are many ways in which the metaphor cannot speak to the vibrancy of life as we know it, but if a vibrant life is a spiritual life, perhaps Guenther's conclusion is inescapable.

My wife had planned very carefully to have a natural birth, which meant, among other things, that there would be no pain medication. In order to accomplish her plan, she enlisted the help of midwives.

Midwives are a different kind of healthcare provider in today's world. It is difficult to contrast them to other providers, because no one would disagree with them outright. They believe that the body functions quite well normally, although there are rare exceptions. They try to normalize birth as a human event, and less of a medical crisis. Tone is everything. It is hard to typify the character of a midwife. Like many women, they are strong, but the courage and confidence of the midwife are remarkably inspiring. And that's not an accident—she needs to be inspiring, and that confidence is one of many preinterventions to make sure things are set up for success.

At my daughter's birth, we were also assisted by a doula, which is Greek for "servant." She is there to support, and she did many of the things that are traditionally connected with midwifery. She was able to help get what my wife needed, and she had an implicit understanding of what those needs might be. It might be food, water, sometimes a shoulder to lean on, or even counterpressure on the back. Perhaps most importantly, she knew what to say, although our midwife also had a way with words. Words were very important.

It may also be helpful to emphasize that although I was there, and it was necessary that I be there, there were so many ways in which I could not step into the midwifery role. I wasn't the midwife, I was the husband. It may even be the case that a mother prefers to rely solely on her mate—I'm sure that happens. I'm sure that there are many husbands out there who may be more helpful than I was, more experienced and able to do some of those things. Some, but not all.

But one of the things that I saw there as husband was that the role of midwife is necessarily *particular and exclusive*. Midwifing is a very specific

---

1. Guenther, *Holy Listening*, loc. 1017–19.

The Midwife

way of standing next to someone, and it excludes other ways of being. It is adaptable, yes, in our case our doula and midwife had to complement each other because each would normally have operated differently in the absence of the other. But adaptable or not, to be someone's midwife is to know them in a unique kind of way. The entire relationship is contextualized around one purpose; a purpose that any two people will experience very differently.

So what follows are a few observations that are true of midwives in general. Some of these may seem repetitive, but each carries a special nuance.

It is utterly implicit that the *midwife does not have the most important job*. It is crucial to remain clear about where the locus of accomplishment lies. Midwives try very hard, but they are not "laboring." Human beings are very resilient and capable of tremendous change. In spiritual midwifery, the locus of agency rests in the one who is mothering, and not in the "expertise" of the helping professional. Socrates makes this abundantly clear. He says in the *Thaeatetus*, "My art of midwifery is in general like theirs; the only difference is that my patients are men, not women, and my concern is not with the body but with the soul that is in the travail of birth. . . . But the delivery is heaven's work . . . ."[2] Socrates is only a partner involved in a much bigger drama.

While the midwife is not the one doing the principal work, there is such a thing as a good midwife or even an inexperienced midwife. *The good midwife is the one you don't notice.* The midwife is an important position, and those skills require practice and development. Spiritual midwifery puts the practice into practical theology.

The birthing process is fundamentally dynamic. Movement and trajectory are a lot more important than pathology and diagnosis. Midwives are not detached analysts; they are engaged catalysts. Most of the skills and interventions they have are about movement and restoring the motion of the soul. All effort is directed toward facilitating movement—it's not about finding an answer and it's certainly not about getting someone else to agree. Everything is directed toward the dynamic process.

A tension emerges here in the writing. The paradox arises to where I need to try to describe transition to the uninitiated without defining transition for those who have experiences of their own.

---

2. Quoted in Kierkegaard, *Concluding Unscientific Postscript*, 279n.

Part I—Poetics, Aesthetics, and Ethics

More than "agents of change"—which has become cliché—midwives are *guides through transition*. Transition can be the most frightening and disorienting part of the natural and unmedicated birth process and it is so unnerving that no one would choose an experience like that. Physically speaking, the body changes its entire work of opening to the work of birthing the baby. For a moment, the body seems untrustworthy and that is terrifying. Midwives, therefore, assume the responsibility of leading others through life's greatest transitions.

In her groundbreaking work *Holy Listening*, Margaret Guenther spends an entire chapter embellishing and translating the midwife and birth metaphor as it relates to spiritual midwifery. She writes:

> The first stage of labor ends in a period of transition, which can be frightening, even terrifying if it is unexpected. Even when the transition is understood, it is of surprising power. The birthgiver is gripped by tremendous force and feels that she has somehow lost control. Everything is suddenly too big and too powerful. All the weeks of careful preparation and instruction seem inadequate and trivial. The birthgiver had thought she was prepared and "knew just what to do"—and now it doesn't work! She might even feel betrayed: no one has told her the truth, or perhaps no one has previously confronted and understood the truth.[3]

The chaos and confusion here are organic; it's not the confounding from without but the terror from within. What's helpful here is how Guenther translates this to the spiritual life. She says, "In the birth process, the dark, seemingly chaotic period of transition is the time of greatest discomfort and—at least from the birthgiver's viewpoint—greatest need for the supportive presence of the midwife. In our spiritual lives, too, it is a pivotal time. The old ways no longer serve."[4]

It is worth noting that theologian Karen Hanson concurs: "One of the first things a midwife must learn is *what travail looks like!* And, seeing it, not to shrink from it."[5] Here, she is using the biblical term to describe the part of childbirth that is so frightening. It is this old notion of travail that is so organic to transition.

What is crucial here is to see the value of good midwifery. The timing could not be more important. This is a hard time and true help is needed.

---

3. Guenther, *Holy Listening*, loc. 1205–8.
4. Ibid., loc. 1208–11.
5. Hanson, "The Midwife," 206.

"The lonely times of transition can be terrible, for they are times of spiritual homelessness."[6] Even when things go well, support is needed. "One of the unwelcome surprises of transition is the sense of loss that inevitably accompanies self-transcendence and new growth."[7]

Midwives are prepared and they have enough experience to understand what people need. This could really be two points. By being prepared, midwives have already set things up for success. Many dangerous things are avoided before they ever gets to the level of danger. Beyond that, they have enough experience with the territory to know what people are likely to need. Some of the work may require give-and-take, but there will also be points where guidance is necessary. As with so many specialties in healthcare, patients cannot be expected to self-diagnose. They can report experiences of pain and that communication is required for good healthcare, but they need the guidance and expertise of the midwife.

An experienced midwife is very powerful. *While they do have skills and techniques to draw on, they also know how to get out of the way.* A lot of their expertise lies in blending in with the background. It is assumed that people are capable and empowered.

From the perspective of spiritual direction, Margaret Guenther put it this way:

> The midwife is present to another in a time of vulnerability, working in areas that are deep and intimate. It is a relationship of trust and mutual respect. Unlike most physicians, she does not fear that her professionalism will be threatened by a degree of intimacy with the women who have come to her for help. She is willing to be called by her given name, even as she addresses the birthgiver by hers. She does things with, not to, the person giving birth.[8]

Jesus and Socrates

In studying spiritual midwifery and spiritual rebirth, there are two major sources with whom we need to dialogue from the West: Jesus and Socrates. The first question is, if they are both talking about spiritual midwifery, and

---

6. Guenther, *Holy Listening*, loc. 1215–16.
7. Ibid., loc. 1252–53.
8. Ibid., loc. 1042–45.

Part I—Poetics, Aesthetics, and Ethics

if their practice of it is similar to each other, are they in some way talking to each other? What is the relationship between Socrates and Jesus?

There are some token similarities in the lives of the two men. Both were famous teachers and neither wrote anything down. They were also both executed by the state, for controversial teachings on the nature of piety, corrupting the youth, and general disruption of the state. In very rough analogy, both of these men sacrificed their lives for the sake of an idea. But can we do any better than these generalities?

We know that the two movements have influenced each other. Early Christianity relied on the apparatus of Greek thought for the evolution of its theology. And we also know that subsequent movements in philosophy, such as that of the Neoplatonists, were also important in the overall history of Christianity. But was there any earlier connection?

Hard to say. Jesus and Socrates were about 400 years apart. Jesus lived around the Jordan region and Socrates was halfway across the Mediterranean in Athens. We know that through Alexander Greek culture had spread much farther than the Sea of Galilee and that there are plenty of other people farther from Athens than Jesus who were familiar with Socrates. We also know that Jesus was an excellent student and was quickly recognized as a teacher, though we don't know the details of his education. The historical record shows that Jesus was very familiar with the stories and texts of the Jewish tradition, but there is never any kind of direct reference to Socrates or anything else, for that matter, that might be associated with secular philosophy.

But even though there are a lot of questions that can never be answered, one fact remains unshakable: both Socrates and Jesus relied heavily on the metaphor of the spiritual rebirth.

As it turns out, there is a passage in John—and only in John—that holds the metaphor (John 3:1–21). Jesus is talking to his friend Nicodemus about the spiritual kingdom and says the only way to enter it is to be born again. That sounded very familiar. Socrates said that he saw himself as a spiritual midwife. In the *Theaetetus*, he says that his "concern is not with the body but with the soul that is in the travail of birth."[9] Jesus, on the other hand, is talking about the experience of spiritual transformation and what that feels like for the one who is transformed. It's like being born again. That image was so powerful that there is an entire branch of Christianity that defines itself in terms of being born again. Socrates takes this metaphor

---

9. Quoted in Kierkegaard, *Concluding Unscientific Postscript*, 279n.

from the other side of the dialogical relationship. Socrates talks about what it's like to be a spiritual midwife. Both Jesus and Socrates seem to suggest that the person giving birth and the person being born again are one in the same.

Just to be clear and accurate, Jesus uses the metaphor of "born again" once, but also references the "time of travail" and "birth pangs" (John 3:3, John 16:21, Mark 13:8, Matt 24:8). Most of all, the rhetorical structure of spiritual midwifery is a structure that Jesus uses throughout the Gospel of John. This is a favored methodology. It's also helpful to emphasize that this metaphor occurs only in the Gospel of John. John is a philosophical writer from the same hometown as Heraclitus—Ephesus. John seems to borrow the idea of the Logos from Heraclitus. Both John and Socrates were influenced by Heraclitus. While certainties about Jesus and Socrates will always be hidden, it does seem that there was a very, very early relationship between the two movements that followed.

Heraclitus is an enigmatic figure, and tradition has given him the moniker "Heraclitus the Obscure." There are few remaining details about his life, so many of its secrets buried by history. But it's important to appreciate that the term has more to do with the mysterious and mystical nature of his teachings rather than his lack of notoriety; Heraclitus, indeed, is the archetypical riddle wrapped in the enigma.

Heraclitus and Midwifery

By birth, Heraclitus had the rare opportunity, limited only to nobles, to get involved in Ephesian government. But for some reason he chose not to. He chose to withdraw to the hills outside the city. Disgruntled by the problems of society, he became a hermit and developed his teachings. Some of these teachings were written down and have survived through quotation.

The impact of his teaching is significant even if remains "obscure." For one thing, Heraclitus said the Divine Spirit was like fire. Like other cosmologists, Heraclitus envisioned the Immortal Principle in elemental terms. The Immortal Principle is ever-burning. Fire also appealed to Heraclitus because of its dynamic properties. Flickering flames are always changing, even as they change other things. He says, "All things equally exchange for fire as does fire for all things."[10] Fire brings heat and illumination. Fire cooks as well as consumes. Fire then becomes the essence of all transaction. Fire and heat are the

---

10. Quoted in Geldard, *Remembering Heraclitus*, 158.

dominant metaphors in Heraclitus's work. It is immeasurable to what extent Heraclitus influenced later Christian terminology of the Holy Spirit, where in the Pentecost story the Holy Spirit is also depicted by flames.

Heraclitus is also credited for introducing the concept of the logos to the West. The logos is the ancestor of logic, as the name suggests. It is often translated as "word." When John begins his gospel, "In the beginning was the Word," the term that actually occurs there is *logos*. Apparently, John saw fit to tie his understanding of the incarnation of Jesus with the older Greek notion of the logos. John's analogy, of course, is brilliant. Back in Genesis, in the beginning God creates the world by speaking, saying "Let there be light, let there be dry land," and so on. John takes it up a notch. John says that God spoke, yes, and the Word was God and the Word was with God. Then the Word became flesh and dwelt among us. The logos, says John, is none other than Jesus Christ. This transitive equation of Jesus and God anticipated the later concept of the Trinity by at least a hundred years.

The association of John and Heraclitus is not an accident. The patron deity of Ephesus was Artemis, hunter goddess and twin of Apollo. In some stories, she was a fertility goddess and a moon goddess. As was the custom, Heraclitus would have deposited his writings at the temple of Artemis. The temple no longer exists today, but it served as a cultural center of such fame that it brought Ephesus to global prominence. Five hundred years later, John had access to Heraclitus's writings. John was from Ephesus, wrote there, and would have easy access to Heraclitus's philosophy.

Socrates was much closer to Heraclitus than John was, only a generation apart. The Athenian held the Ephesian in high esteem. When asked what he thought of Heraclitus, Socrates said that he liked what he understood, but that he would need to be a Delian diver to really get to the bottom of it. The Delians were known to be deep-sea divers.

It's hard to find Socrates's commentary on Heraclitus, so this is an important nugget. This might be misattributed or a favorite colloquial expression of the time, but scholars are quick to point out that this is a superlative remark coming from Socrates. The Oracle at Delphi had pronounced Socrates the wisest man in Athens. Legend has it that the secret to Socrates's wisdom was that he knew that he didn't know anything, as opposed to all the experts of the day that thought they knew everything. For the man whose wisdom is a kind of holy ignorance, what Socrates is alleged to have said can only be seen as superlative praise.

The Midwife

The metaphor of spiritual midwifery is a key shared term between Socrates and Jesus. It's a metaphor with so much traction that it catches on and defines the Jesus movement (note again that, to this day, many Christians define their spirituality in terms of being born again), even though the metaphor only appears in one of the four Gospels. What's more, the metaphor also conveys the similar rhetorical technology that is employed in the dialogues of Socrates and Jesus. The irony of Socrates helps makes a lot of sense out of the mystical parables of Jesus.

Further, the influence of Heraclitus is a powerful connection between classical Greek philosophy and Christianity. In the same pericope where Socrates describes himself as a midwife, he reverences the goddess Artemis. Throughout the dialogues of Plato, Socrates references and reverences many gods and goddesses in accordance with the theme. What's important to realize here is that by alluding to Artemis, Socrates places himself in the school of Heraclitus, who had deposited his writings in the temple dedicated to her.

The strong fingerprint of Heraclitus in both the Gospel of John and Socrates's statement on midwifery is another confirmation that we are right to consult both Jerusalem and Athens.

Summary of the Midwife

- The role of midwife is necessarily particular and exclusive.
- It is utterly implicit that the midwife does not have the most important job.
- The good midwife is the one you don't notice.
- The birthing process is fundamentally dynamic. More than "agents of change"—which has become cliché—midwives are guides through transition.
- Midwives are prepared and have enough experience to understand what people need.
- While they do have techniques to draw on, they also know how to get out of the way.
- Spiritual midwifery rests on a set of philosophical and theological ideas that weave through John, Heraclitus, Jesus, and Socrates.

Chapter 2

The Baby

> You would not find out the limits of the soul,
> even by traveling every path,
> so deep a Logos does it have.
>
> HERACLITUS

THE SUCCESS OF THIS project rests in a riddle wrapped in the proverbial enigma. If spiritual midwifery is about helping someone else through the process of spiritual rebirth, who or what is the baby? For that matter, who or what is giving birth?

As it turns out, in our parlance, the very person giving birth is also the one being reborn. While the midwife stands outside that relationship, the one being reborn is clearly engaged in both locations of the birth metaphor.

So, this may create some questions. For starters, what are we saying is being born? The psychological self? The true self? Are any of these the product of this process?

To a large extent, it becomes counterproductive to hammer out definitive answers to these questions. After all, we are ultimately trying to explore a multivalent metaphor, with layers and layers of depth and meaning. We are not trying to create a static and dead allegory where each aspect of the poetic image has a unique and specific referent. This is not some kind of gnostic code to be cracked as a secret map to a hidden cosmology.

The Baby

People go through a significant process of change that certain religions and philosophies have described as being reborn. And even though it is obvious that in the world as we know it one could never be born by oneself, just as one could never birth oneself, there is enough descriptive truth to the metaphor that some of the aspects of being born and some of the aspects of giving birth equally apply.

There are also some theological resonances here. There are many people who equate this kind of rebirth with the theological work of soteriology, where this kind of rebirth is the prescription for successful transition to the afterlife. Categorically, I would gently recommend resisting those kinds of equations and formulas, at least insofar as we want to remain true to our exploration of spiritual midwifery. This understanding of midwifery is not a suitable vehicle for the establishment of complicated doctrine. At the same time, I want to reinforce a commitment to being theologically friendly, not theologically averse. Even for Christians who believe that being reborn is the single requirement to eternal life, I think they would agree that life everlasting is a qualitative change that begins in this life. If we find everlasting life, it begins now. If we drink from ever living water, the quenching begins now. It is that experience of now where Jesus lived and where we work in the care of souls. In this context of now is where we want to explore process and movement, especially spiritual movement. For readers who immediately collapse language of rebirth with salvation, I'd like to focus the attention on the transformation that is experienced in this life.

Further, I want to guard against an equally static psychological interpretation. If we think of the self as some kind of destination of personality, sort of the culmination of self-actualization, that is also a different kind of formula which also needs to be resisted.

Problems with the Soul

In Western philosophy, the concept of "the soul" has not been doing so well. Many people don't even believe that the soul exists. And maybe this is symptomatic of where we are at the end of the world; no one believes in God or the soul, and all things spiritual have come into doubt. On the face of it, maybe doubt in God is understandable. God is the greatest of all mysteries that defy comprehension. We can never prove that God exists and the universe seems to be designed that way. Part of the nature of reality includes secrets.

Part I—Poetics, Aesthetics, and Ethics

On the other hand, if souls exist, we are the living proof and there is an inundation of evidence. This is both tragic and comic—we no longer believe in ourselves. We believe in our desires, but we no longer see the self as the sacred vessel of faith. The self and the importance of the individual have become a joke. Everything has been academically deconstructed. It is no longer a given that there is a world of meaning beyond our own impressions and mistaken perceptions. At the risk of becoming a traditionalist curmudgeon, I do not think it is an accident that we no longer believe in the soul, as I am reminded of Freud's universal truth: the self desires to remain unconscious.

It doesn't help that Scripture itself is vague on the subject of the soul, perhaps because something as obvious as the soul didn't require explanation. Scripture of course references the human soul and spirituality, but is short on the kinds of academic definitions to which we are so accustomed. In short, Scripture does not spell it out—there are holy things about which it prefers to not speak. The problem seems to be complicated by our attempts to put things into words. Ever since Descartes's famous "I think, therefore I am," we have been struggling to name the soul. In Western thought, we have followed Descartes's trajectory by seeking to locate the soul in rationality.

This is really the crux of it. Once philosophy became enamored with rationalism, it became harder and harder to do meaningful work with concepts of the soul. At one point philosophy and religion nourished each other. That relationship has been breaking down for a long time, and one of the wedge points has been the concept of the soul.

There are a few underlying complications with this methodology; there are some ways that this spiritual quest in the material world was ruined from the get-go. Rationality has sought to find the physiological seat of the soul. Where is the soul? If we think that our intellect is our soul, then the most likely place is the brain—or even some precise region of it, a piece of it, some holy part. If we say that the soul is the measurable mind, that is, the brain, then we are saying that the soul cannot survive death. Because one way that the question of the soul has been answered in the West has been to say that for all intents and purposes, the soul is the brain—no immortality. One downside of this is the entire concept of the soul is reduced to one cerebral organ.

The other move has been to say that the soul has nothing to do with the mind. The soul is not the body, or any part of it. This has led to the

The Baby

conclusion that there is some kind of immaterial consciousness that is a part of our life on earth and that experiences the world somehow, but because of its very immateriality, it is not subject to the same forces of life and death that circumscribe the world we know. The problem is that any concept of the soul that is so categorically distinct from anything tangible has no way of engaging the world—none whatsoever.

These two extremes merge together to form a paradox, and a paradox that makes it hard to have any kind of working model of the soul. On the one hand, we are talking about a soul that is a physical thing in a physical body—and as with any other part of the body, vulnerable to the experience of death. On the other hand, we are talking about the existence of something so removed from the reality of life that it has no way to interact with life as we know it. With both of these conditions, it is difficult to maintain that there is a living soul that interacts with the world and is capable of some kind of immortality. The contemporary, rational mind has framed the question and the definition of the soul in such a way that it cannot possibly be resolved. The conscious mind then remains in this thoughtful universe all by itself, which is perhaps what it wanted all along.

Both of these problems stem from the same source: trying to define the soul as a fixed, unmoving, and eternal kernel of being. It is easy to attribute this to Descartes, because this is how we have learned to tell the story of the history of our rationalism, but the ideas behind the ideas go back to the foundations of our civilization. These ideas run through the history of Western Christianity. They run back through the natural philosophy of Aquinas, back through Augustine, and all the way back to Aristotle. And all of these thinkers have approached the question in this way: if there really is a self, then it must have some kind of substance, and if that substance is not limited by the laws of nature, then it must be eternal.

But maybe not. Maybe there is a soul that is capable of experiencing eternity, but is not a physical place in the body. Maybe there is an idea of the soul that is capable of flux, flexibility, and change.

What if the soul exists, but we have been looking for it in all the wrong places? What if we can't find it in a body part (people once thought that the soul was the heart, or even the liver), because it's not a part at all, but rather the unique set of relationships *between* the parts that make us human? Perhaps what we call the soul is a cluster of sacred relationships. This cluster of relationships is unique and is more or less self-aware.

Part I—Poetics, Aesthetics, and Ethics

The Dynamic Soul

While it is helpful for the midwife to think of the soul as a living cluster of sacred relationships, it is not necessary. This possible model of the soul is remote and abstract, and the terms it uses may be wrong. The truth is that we don't have access to the divine language and we are not able to name these things definitively. Socrates suggests that we are limited to approximations and metaphor. And Scripture tells countless stories where God keeps silent on a great many things and the greatest of all is the very name of the divine. We are never given that name.[1]

However, there are two ramifications of conceiving of the soul in this way that are necessary for midwifery, and they deserve identification. For the midwife, the soul is first and foremost dynamic. The soul is constantly changing, moving, growing. And suddenly we are struck by the obvious nature of this truth: every living thing is changing, moving, and growing. That's what it means to be alive, and somehow all those historical attempts to define the soul apart from dynamic change seem problematic from the start. If we are talking about a living thing that seems to survive physical death, it would have to have at least some traits of other living things.

The second such ramification is that the soul is fundamentally relational. Again, this seems sort of obvious. If human beings are intended for some kind of relationship with the divine, then they ought to be inherently equipped for relationship. But it goes a little deeper than the obvious. They are equipped for relationship because what they *are* is relationship. Wholes are undeniably greater than the sum of their parts, but wholes could never be diametrically opposite their parts. Human being could not be so utterly suited for relationship if it wasn't as much in the core of their being as their own DNA.

---

1. While I think this is a true enough fact to build on, I acknowledge that many readers may disagree. There are many places in Scripture where God is revealed, but I don't believe that revelation to be exhaustive. Certainly, for Christians the Gospels are revelation embodied. But to let go of all mystery is a dangerous hermeneutic, one which could easily destroy Trinitarian thought. Much of midwifery happens in the white space on the page, beyond the limits of language. And the belief that language is both created and limited is a theological idea to which we will continually return. Since Adam, language and naming are tied to mastery and dominion. And in the way that the tetragrammaton is not pronounced by the pious, we might well remember that part of the reason why the face of God is hidden is for our protection. I like how Heraclitus says it: "The one, the only wisdom does and yet does not consent to be called Zeus" (Geldard, *Remembering Heraclitus*, 159). God has never asked to be called "God," and yet many of us do so. God is merciful and free, and we can call God whatever we want. But that doesn't mean we should.

So the soul is both dynamic and relational; at least, that's how the midwife sees it. And the midwife needs to see it that way, because most of the work of the midwife deals with various relationships and spiritual dynamics, often exploring difficult relationships to restore movement of the soul, or in looking at how dynamics shape or impact core relationships. If the midwife is going to give help that is needful and relevant, there needs to be a basic familiarity of the what and the how. What is it, and how does it move?

It is helpful to anticipate that there is a logos here, that there is a *telos* to this process. Psychology begs the question: what is the psyche? But let us not forget that the psyche is on a trajectory, a path, and this logos is going somewhere, becoming something.

While both Jesus and Socrates talk about the soul, neither is exceedingly forthcoming on what exactly it is. Even though Socrates philosophizes freely about the soul he is not able (or perhaps, more wisely, unwilling) to dissect and diagram the parts of the soul. That said, it is more than noteworthy that his most famous argument for the immortality of the soul is not its intangibility (an argument that says the soul is fundamentally immaterial and therefore immune to entropy and death), but rather, the prevenient motion of the soul. Whether or not that argumentation is compelling to the rationalist's paradox, it does cement the interpretation that Socrates saw the soul as dynamic. And so much of Jesus' message and tone seems to be predicated on a similar belief; so much of what he says bids us to move, to draw hither, to take an action, to resume a spiritual journey that was left some time ago.

As to the relational piece, there is an irrefutable amount of data that both men valued relationship to the utmost. Both men lived their lives pursing relationships around them, and both men died their deaths for a greater belief in relationship. And specifically with regard to Jesus, it is only through the hope of a divine relationship that the Jesus movement comes into focus and meaning at all.

Models of the Soul

It is one thing to say that the human soul exists as a cluster of sacred relationships, but relationships between what and what? How do we understand them?

We may never be able to fully delineate them. However, there have been many models throughout history that allow for a dynamic soul that is relational. Ultimately, we can't prove or rationalize which model is correct, but we can affirm that this has been a traditional way to think about the soul.

Christian Scripture seems to suggest some basic dynamics. When the Law requires that we love God with all our heart, soul, and strength (Deut 6:5), the Law suggests that there are three modalities—or at least capacities—of the human person. Indeed, Jesus summarizes this commandment, sometimes substituting "mind" for "strength," or leaving the tripartite formula altogether for the collective four terms (Mark 12:30). While these terms are not specifically defined in the text, they still suggest a model of a dynamic self which consists of several interrelated parts. Tradition is firm that the self cannot be reduced to one of these modalities, and that there is a dynamism between these parts that is partially comprehensible but ultimately unknowable by empiricism.

Kierkegaard on the Soul

One of the most thoughtful possibilities for a working model of the soul comes from Danish theologian Søren Kierkegaard.[2] And we shall see that Kierkegaard has a lot to say about spiritual midwifery. He suggests that the self is a series of dialectical relationships.

The soul, for Kierkegaard, consists of three relationships. One relationship exists between what the Dane calls "Possibility" and "Necessity." Human beings are capable agents and they can do things and make choices. In this sense, they participate in Possibility, and there's a lot that they can do. But they can't do everything. And more to the point, they have all kinds of limits—limits that stem directly from the human condition and limits that they find in their environments. Gravity is one of those limits, and so is mortality.

Another relationship is a reflexive relationship—your relationship to yourself. This is the birth of consciousness. After all, there are many living things that exist in the continuum between Possibility and Necessity. But we also have the recognition that we are here. And we have complicated relationships to the person we were in the past, and we plan ahead for the

---

2. Kierkegaard's model for the soul is most clearly described in *Sickness Unto Death*.

person we are going to be in the future. We also have a myriad of feelings about who we are in the present.

Kierkegaard's final relationship exists between our self and God. There are different dimensions to this. We relate to the divine Person that we think God is, and we project all manner of values and beliefs onto that Person. We think that God approves of this, and disapproves of that, but much of what we project is likely to come out of our own values—or worse: our own self-deception. This isn't any different from the other inner relationships of the soul. We are just as likely to relate to a false sense of ourselves as a false sense of who God is. But projections aside, we also have a true relationship to the God that actually exists even though much of God's experience of this relationship is veiled in mystery. Each of these relationships are dialectical. A soul consists of all three of these relationships. If any one of these relationships is dysfunctional, then that can cause problems for the whole person. Part of the attractiveness of Kierkegaard's model is the dialectical dynamism (still tripartite) that speaks to the human condition from a recognizably existential perspective.

It might be helpful to explain why dialectical thought is especially inducive for midwifery. When things are considered dialectically, they are immediately assumed to be in relationship to one another. Sometimes the relationship is one of polar opposites. Sometimes the relationship can be understood as a continuum. Sometimes the two elements paradoxically cancel each other out so that they both can't be true at the same time. Sometimes, it's all of the above. Dialectical thought emphasizes three things: the two that are linked somehow, and the relationship between. Indeed, in dialectical thinking, it's often that *tertium quid* that's the most powerful idea of all.

Socrates

The centerpiece of the dialogue *Phaedrus* is Socrates's theory of the soul. Socrates says that the soul is like a chariot driver. There are two horses that pull this chariot. One horse is good and the other is bad. The good horse is a noble, white horse. The white horse is obedient and ever-attentive to the driver. The bad horse is a black horse, and this horse is passionate and unruly. This horse refuses to cooperate and only wants to do its own thing.

Traditional interpretation has wanted to understand Socrates as uplifting the intellectual and rational and denigrating the emotional. Plato

Part I—Poetics, Aesthetics, and Ethics

was Socrates's greatest interpreter, and Plato started the large project of the Academy, and perhaps it was important to him to assert the primacy of reason. If Plato's project was the intellectual Academy, then he took for its mascot the white horse of Socrates.

But this isn't what Socrates said. Socrates said that the soul is like the chariot driver, not the white horse. The two horses, after all, are only horses. What counts is the driver. Here is the influence of Heraclitus.

Heraclitus came before Socrates, and it seems that Socrates was influenced by him. One of the core attributes of Heraclitus's thought is the role of dialectical tension. Heraclitus also emphasized the importance of change and motion, and reflecting on Heraclitus allows us to reexamine the parable about these horses. Maybe the philosophical tradition had its own reasons for backing the white horse, but the parable is clear. The chariot driver is the harmony of the dialectical tension. There are always going to be opposites. What counts are the choices we make between them. That's where we find out who we are.

This is not the "Allegory of the Two Horses," as Plato would have us believe. This is the "Parable of the Chariot Driver."

Socrates is talking about the soul, offering depth of insight that we don't see again in Western thought the emergence of Freud. Freud has a very similar model for the soul. Instead of a white horse, Freud offers the Superego—the innate sense of what we should do, what we ought to do, at any given moment. Instead of the black horse, Freud talks about the Id as the seat of unrestrained desire. Between them is the Ego, constantly resolving these eternal internal conflicts as we engage the world around us. Just how deep are Socrates' insights? In a way, Socrates anticipates the entire development of psychology.[3] Psychology itself is the logos and language of the psyche and soul.

---

3. This is a place where psychology has much to bring to the conversation. Academic philosophy has left religion with models of the soul that are basically fixed and unchanging for eternity. Psychology, on the other hand, has been embracing models of the self that are very dialectical and dynamic. The Myers-Briggs Type Indicator is basically a model of the self organized around four dichotomies. Are these dichotomies more useful or complete than Kierkegaard's? That's fair to debate, but psychology nonetheless has been understanding the self in this dynamic way.

The Baby

Final Thoughts

There is no one, complete model for the soul. It's probably not even desirable that there would be one. If there was only one, that discussion would become rigid and unhelpfully static. The limits of human language would only make a definitive model worse, as undoubtedly some very important dimensions of personhood would be eclipsed and overlooked. Spiritual midwifery works best with models that emphasize relationship and the dynamic movement of the soul.

Our purpose here has been to clarify the subject of our inquiry, not to define it. We are working with the soul, even though we will never be completely able to say what the soul is. We have also sought to acknowledge that the conversation about the soul between philosophy and religion has run aground, but there are numerous dynamic models of the soul all across the theological spectrum (and even psychology) that might give the conversation flight again.

Chapter 3

Medicine and Dialogue

SOCRATES:
Rhetoric is like medicine.

PHAEDRUS:
How so?

SOCRATES:
Why, because medicine has to define the nature of the body and rhetoric of the soul . . . .

PHAEDRUS:
There, Socrates, I suspect that you are right.

SOCRATES:
. . . The rhetorician, who teaches his pupil to speak scientifically, will particularly set forth the nature of that being to which he addresses his speeches;
and this, I conceive, to be the soul.
. . . His whole effort is directed to the soul for in that he seeks to produce conviction . . . .

PHAEDRUS:
Yes.

SOCRATES:
Then clearly . . . any one . . . who teaches rhetoric in earnest will give an exact description of the nature of the soul.

Medicine and Dialogue

Dialogue is the medium for midwifery, the vessel for this *via media*, the ultimate container for conversation. Dialogue is where it all happens. Dialogue is not just the fruitful exchange between persons, but in the very best sense of the Platonic tradition, we see that human discourse has the potential to touch the divine.

In general, human religion and spirituality are very aware of connections, attachments, and relationships. Even more, there is something intrinsic to Christianity that always wants to bring the Christian into conversation with others. Conversation is not the same thing as conversion, but as you might suspect, their etymologies are a tangled mess. There is a spectrum of witness that spans human possibility for the sublime at the one end and the inhumane at the either; at one end we find Jesus' simple recognition that someone needs to talk, and at the other we find those being compelled to convert under violence. So there are admittedly numerous failures where the conversation has been corrupted, but from the very beginning there was an awareness that a mere conversation has the power to change lives.

There is nothing so daring as dialogue, nothing as daunting as submitting yourself to the gauntlet of the opinions of another. When we expose ourselves to dialogue we are surrendering the monologue of our own ego, our own narcissism. A dialogue can go anywhere; that's the beauty of it. But that's also the horror of it. If the dialogue can honestly go anywhere, then that means we have given up control of it, because the only way to know where it's going is to control it. But we give up control, and we give up certainty in this encounter with the other. And if we truly submit to that experience, we will find ourselves changed in the process, for we have exposed the monotony of our consciousness to the music of another.

Our Cultural Model for Dialogue

Developing a working definition of "dialogue" is easier said than done. It's probably better to think of it as an "ethic of dialogue" or "dialogical ethics," or better still, "dialogical hermeneutics."

The deceptive factor is that there are many conversations that are initiated all the time—conversations that have no interest in honest dialogue. Yes, there are two people that are talking to each other. And to some extent, they are hearing each other; that is, they are extremely attentive to the moves of their opponent, but only for the sake of coming up with the better countermove and the best stratagem. There is no genuine vulnerability, no honest engagement; it is conversation in the service of something else and that is usually coercion. The pretense of "mutual dialogue" is only a ruse, a guise to discharge the weapon of verbal coercion at short range. There is no experience of the dialogue as a means of self-transformation; the dialogue is only good for gaining influence over others.

This is also the reason for the failure of political correctness and why it is so intrinsically paradoxical—paradoxical to the point of being so self-contradictory that it was destined for failure. Some people have so much invested in political correctness that they cannot admit that the failure has already happened. They think that the reason that political correctness has not won the day is because there are not enough people that subscribe to it.

Political correctness is actually its own theory of dialogue as expressed by the Western academy. The practice is so pervasive, with the ideas behind it, that a comment or two are required before exploring our own approach to dialogue. A new theory of dialogue must be contrasted to normative ideas that are collectively assumed. We participate in this popular theory of dialogue a dozen times a day. Without necessarily meaning to we conform to its rules and norms even to the point of imposing those rules on others. A deeper appreciation of what dialogue might be calls for a rigorous, even Socratic, examination of this cultural value.

The project of political correctness looks at the cohesion of society as a function of social discourse. If we can get everybody talking together, then the talk itself becomes the social container. That sounds good, right? But then it tries to spell out rules for conducting civil discourse in a civil society. We can say this, but we can't say that. Again, this seems very natural and well-intentioned. If society is merely the network for social discourse, then aren't we going to need some rules for how this discourse is supposed to occur? In the land of democracy, doesn't every effective consensus need a rightful process? One would think so . . .

That's the basic idea. But then it gets complicated. What happens is that people in the throes of discourse get lost in the complexities and the ensuing confusion is the bizarre kind of acrimonious glue that holds everything together; we find ourselves begrudgingly bound by political correctness. At some level we can't help but resent being controlled in our most private recesses of thought. What's more, there is a principle of lowest common denominator at work here, where allegedly we all consent to drop the lowest terms from our vocabulary. But this power to silence becomes its own weapon in the hands of the very human and fallible. We are tempted to destroy one another for the sake of conversational decency.

Political correctness introduces its own terms and virtues, and things like marginalization, inclusivity, diversity, and tolerance circulate in rising currency. But these things are so controversial in themselves that it's never going to be possible to get everyone to agree on how diverse or tolerant we should be. How do we view ourselves without marginalizing anyone? How do we empower the disenfranchised without disenfranchising somebody else? There are some profound questions here, and sadly they never get asked. And so we found ourselves in a culture war at the end of the twentieth century. But the deeper questions can only be suppressed for so long.

As a theory of dialogue, political correctness is simultaneously the means and the ends of Western civilization. It holds the ideal of a peaceful society and the means of getting there. This is where political correctness holds its secret and subversive power. If I can get you into a debate about the merits of political correctness, then in many respects I've already won, because that is precisely the goal of political correctness all along: to engraft an increasing number of participants into this culture-defining metaphor of quasidialogue. But this is also the place where the metaphor fails, because it has no genuine interest in engaging the experience of the other. If the dialogical other experiences the conversation itself as a type of blasphemy, the theory of political correctness has no language to contain that.

It took me a long time to get my mind around this, and I didn't make any progress until I met a high-ranking military chaplain. As he explained to me, we were very interested in stabilizing the Middle East after the original Persian Gulf War. We went over there and employed our very best efforts in the arts of multiculturalism. We did our best to refrain from any offensive speech and we graciously overlooked any exclusivity in the God language displayed by the Islamic interlocutors. They were not impressed. We did not come across as "polite." We came across as godless and holier—or at least superior—than thou.

How could it be any other way? There's no such thing as neutral language. Every kind of grammar is predicated on some type of value system. Trying to completely avoid differences in the name of inclusivity means that inclusivity is more important than identity. It is the substitution of one value for another.

Of course, we didn't need to turn to the Middle East to find this limitation of political correctness. We see this every time political correctness comes into collision with free speech. Every time we say this can't be said and that can't be said, we are negating the possibility of true dialogue. And we don't gain anything by restricting the use of epithets and the expression of deeply held beliefs. We merely require that deeply held beliefs have to be held even deeper. As a result, political correctness has no language for conflict, aside from clichés of "agreeing to disagree," and conflict is a vital part of authentic relationship.

Toward a Theology of Dialogue

There are a few theological and philosophical considerations that are going to help us understand the role of dialogue in midwifery. Jesus and Socrates don't say a lot (but neither do they say nothing) about language, or the sharing of language between persons. Furthermore, beyond anything they are purported to have said, there are two very strong traditions that must irrefutably conclude that Jesus and Socrates used dialogue in a powerful, intentional, and transformative way. There will always be controversy and debate about what they really said, but forever will it be undeniable that they changed the world with their dialogue.

Before we consider these two figures more specifically, it might be helpful to remember what it is that theology, dialogue, and even psychology have in common—and at least linguistically, that is the logos, the term coined by Heraclitus. There is this directive intelligence at work in the universe. That intelligence sears and scores its way into reality, forked and particular, like a strike of lightning across the summer night sky. As Heraclitus says, "The lightning directs everything," and for a moment one thinks fleetingly of Anaxagoras who suggested that *Nous*, or Mind, was the first universal principle.[1] Of course many words are etymologically related, and it is possible to overvalue the ancestry of language. But the reference to the Ephesian is neither unwarranted nor imprecise. Spiritual midwifery comes through the thought of Heraclitus and dialogue is a critical component of midwifery. These ideas are both related and interrelated; they have more than one relation.

To play with the thought of Heraclitus just a bit more, it is fascinating to imagine dialogue as diaLogos, that this logos is living and moving between two persons in conversation, that this logos at the center of our

1. See Geldard, *Remembering Heraclitus*, 158, and Geldard, *Anaxagoras and Universal Mind*.

Medicine and Dialogue

theory is simultaneously at the center of the conversation; that this logos is in fact centering our very selves. Dialogue is not just a location for the application of spiritual midwifery techniques, but rather so much more—it is the embodiment of connection and relationship itself manifested between souls.

Dialogue retains an essentially binary character, that is, it always remains a dialogue—that intrinsic twoness, however many people are engaged in the conversation. We don't call it a trilogue when there are more persons involved and that is because the term is counting the self and the Other (not taking a head count of how many people constitute the Other). As many have said, it is in the experience of the Other, and that larger territory of all Otherness, where we find our very self. This is the ontology of existentialism; we exist against the presence of reality. This is the process of knowing ourselves by our limits. Our very being is the boundary and the beginning of the rest of the world. This is what psychoanalyst Victor Frankl meant when he said, "To exist is to be different" and this is what Robert Pirsig, author of *Zen and the Art of Motorcycle Maintenance*, meant by suggesting that consciousness of all reality is born in the distinction of self and other.[2] In Freudian terms, perhaps, it is the epiphany that there is a mother.

diaLogos and Dialectic

This diaLogos of Heraclitus is particular and defining. It has the power to bifurcate reality like lightning can split the night sky. It is particular and forked, branching here and striking there. And through this powerful particularity, it hits the great watershed of reality dividing all existence into before and after. For a moment, I remember the rage of Dylan Thomas, and his words that fork lightning.

Even though this diaLogos has the vast and expansive power to fraction reality like a sacramental host, its scope is as infinitely deep as it is infinitely wide. When lightning strikes the beach, glass is formed far down the surf. So too does it bore deep into the soul, crystallizing and commanding recesses and resources that we did not even know.

This gets to an even more powerful idea: that of dialectic. Dialectic is one of the oldest and most universal ideas in religion and philosophy. Through dialectic we explore the great contraries and antinomies of life, and nearly all of the religious traditions have this primal idea at their root.

2. Pirsig, *Zen and the Art of Motorcycle Maintenance*.

Part I—Poetics, Aesthetics, and Ethics

What is dialectic? This is not only the subject of another book entirely, but it's the subject of another encyclopedia of inquiry altogether.

So it is hard to wrestle with such an enormous idea so fleetingly, but this is exactly what we must do if our focus is going to remain on spiritual midwifery.

All of the different religious permutations on dialectic revolve around the great polarities and dualities. Sin and grace. Good and evil. Life and death. Male and female. Yin and yang. Creation and destruction. Light and dark. God and Satan. Even being and nonbeing. This is the heart of all dualism. These dualisms capture powerful truths of the particular human experience. We are born into a world of land and water, night and day, cold and heat, and birth and death. Our experience is intensely defined by these polarities.

Dialectical thought embraces all these opposites, but what's more, it also embraces the elastic terrain of the dialectical tension between them. Sometimes, the dialectical approach even embraces what is annihilated or negated by that tension. This is a bit technical, but through the movement around and between these oppositional definitions, it becomes possible to talk about nondualism and where we get into the great religious and philosophical territory of transcendence. Transcendence is that widest of all terrains that is no longer defined by polarities and dualism. In Christianity, Jesus himself becomes the vehicle of transcendence over the realities of sin and death. This could either be religiously, like some spiritual transcendence, or it could be philosophically. Much of what Hegel does with dialectic is around the transcendence of oppositional concepts and philosophies, although it is probably a disservice to Hegel to so starkly define him as categorically philosophical and not religious. But it's not a surprise when Marx comes along and defines dialectic in terms of political philosophy. Simply, many of the most powerful religions and philosophies derive their torque from dialectic.

What's amazing is what Socrates does with it. What Socrates does with dialectic is something I'd like to tie to this growing notion of diaLogos. What happens for Socrates is that the typical oppositions in dialectical thought are manifested and even incarnated by the different players in the dialogue. The great contraries of existence are replaced with conversation partners in a Socratic dialogue, and what emerges out of the dialogue between them then represents the greater transcendence.

Medicine and Dialogue

Two more things. Establishing the metaphor of "spiritual midwifery" in this technique and tradition of the care of souls was not really Socrates's major concern. He was more interested in the work and in the relationships than in its branding for the next two millennia. Recovering that metaphor is a lot more compelling to me than it was to him. He does not describe himself in great detail as a spiritual midwife. There are only a few dialogues where the images and metaphors occur. His term of choice, not for his technique nor for what we call the Socratic method, was for himself, "dialectician." It is thus conclusive that Socrates saw these conversations as an authentic way of engaging the dialectic and its related transcendence.

Further, it is often taught that Socrates is the first philosopher in the West; that those who preceded Socrates were like Heraclitus and Anaxagorus and others (Thales, Pythagorus, and so on). These thinkers are regarded as cosmologists, and generally discounted for the sake of later thinkers following Socrates. The problem with the cosmologists is that they were as much religious thinkers as philosophers, each trying to understand the cosmos in terms of a grand principle (with Heraclitus fire, with Thales water). Socrates, it is taught, delivers philosophy to the study of phenomena and the dawn of rationalism in the West. I'd like to suggest that Socrates was not the beginning of something new as much as the completion and culmination of something very old. I'd like to suggest that Socrates was the last of the cosmologists in the grand tradition and for him the eternal principal was dialectic. The sacrament for dialectic?

Dialogue itself.

Jesus and the Dialogue

The New Testament and Gospels have their own reason for being. Their purpose is not to articulate all that is meant herein by dialogue. Still, considerable emphasis is placed on the speech of Jesus. Dominant themes like teaching, speaking, hearing, verbal authority, dialogical inclusivity, dynamic contradiction (literally, to speak against), and especially parable all vibrate to the passionate pitch of dialogue.

It is no small footnote that John's Jesus is presented as the Word, and even though this is not shared with the rest of the synoptics, the early church councils all embraced the preeminence of the Logos without question. Of course, dialogue cannot happen without words and their exchange. Whatever is meant by John's assertion that a first-century Semitic person

Part I—Poetics, Aesthetics, and Ethics

was present at the creation of the universe, it must include the understanding that this creative Word is central to God's dialogue with humanity. It is the Jewish philosopher Philo who speculates that Heraclitus, in turn, is borrowing his logos from Genesis, where God creates simply by speaking. It is nothing short of this infinite creative power that John says we encounter in the person of Jesus.

Matthew 18:20 expresses a prophetic and political commitment to the value of dialogue. Jesus says, "For where two or three are gathered in my name, there am I in the midst of them." What makes this scandalous is the contrasting concept of the *minyan*, where ten Jews were required to gather together for the creation of specific worship. Numerically speaking Jesus lowers the bar, from ten to two, but simultaneously elevates the value of individual human interaction. The scandal rings twice as loud here, because Matthew is written especially for a Jewish audience. Wherever two or three are gathered, Jesus promises to be the divine *tertium quid*. Furthermore the centrality of collective spirituality is dispersed, perhaps the democratization of divine intimacy. This democratization is no throwaway detail: here we see that the religious community is subordinate to the dialogical relationship. The life of the community is always an essential feature of corporate religion, and to threaten the vitality of the community in this way is no less revolutionary today, as mainline Christian denominations find themselves in numerical decline. Interestingly, the number is preserved at two—no less—and we get a scriptural hint of the need for confession as well as a confessional partner, and the sacramental quality that characterizes those pastoral encounters.

These few paragraphs in no way exhaust the wealth of the subject. The interested reader is encouraged to revisit the conversations of Jesus. Each manifestation of dialogue has something unique to reveal. Still, it may be helpful to acknowledge one trait of Jesus' dialogues that is often counterintuitive. *Indirect communication is an authentic vehicle for dialogue.* This might be shocking. For some, it can be hard to imagine that Jesus would be anything other than completely transparent, but his "transparency" is a questionable virtue. It is questionable because it can fuse the value of honesty with the experience of immediacy and spontaneity—perhaps a lack of intentionality. It is possible to have responses that are skillful and purposeful without any loss of honesty. It is possible to speak powerfully with life-giving words, even if those words are vulnerable to misunderstanding. There is no reason to lock this observation into a theological framework, but for those readers who bring a theological reference to Jesus, those beliefs only serve to intensify and magnify the observation. Whatever it was that God was trying to achieve in the work and person of Jesus Christ, it was not so important that Jesus felt it necessary to give up the value of indirect communication. Rather, however far God reached across the cosmos into the life of Jesus the message was so important that it could only be entrusted in this indirect way.

Whatever the parables are, "transparent" they are not. Moreover, even when Jesus is trying very hard to be explicit, there is very little real understanding on the other side. So if "transparency" is some kind of judgment about the effectiveness of communication, it becomes harder to build the case that Jesus shared that particular value. Dialogue can move in very intentional ways that defy the unstructured nature of casual conversation.

Socrates and the Dialogue

One of the most overwhelming pieces of data from the Socratic record is the complete permeation of the missional spirit that typifies the Socratic dialogue. The edifices of Plato's thought are neither the theses nor the theories, and not even the philosophies, but *The Dialogues*. Each one of these texts is a resounding testament to just how important dialogue was to Socrates.

To explore the idea a bit further, there are places where Socrates directly references elements of dialogue itself—perhaps some aspect of conversation or some theory of language (under the category of rhetoric, for instance). Socrates explores the philosophy of dialogue with great precision, complexity, and sophistication (as in the cases where Socrates expounds the dialectical method or what it means to be a dialectician). But the most pervasive concept of dialogue emanates from his use of philosophy as project. Yes, Socrates talks about philosophical subjects all the time, but in terms of philosophy as a verb, philosophy as something to do, what Socrates is really doing is dialogue itself. And what it means to do philosophy is to enter into a conversation with another, a lifelong conversation that never ends. When Socrates is trying to missionize—even evangelize—the people of Athens into a life of philosophy, what he's really trying to do is pull people into the great never-ending dialogue. Whatever Plato's given text is about, the volume itself is a monument to its namesake, *The Dialogues*.

Jesus and Socrates both expressed a radical commitment to dialogue. Not only did they spend the very currency of their lives, on a daily basis, experiencing the sacredness of conversation and connection, but they also very clearly chose to die for the things they said. And for each, even though the content often reached the divine and sublime, it is important to appreciate that they didn't die for an utterance or a theory, but they died for the sake of the underlying relationship where the dialogue occurs. Both Jesus and Socrates had ample opportunities to try to talk their way out of a death sentence. Socrates even has the opportunity to mount an escape before drinking the hemlock, but it was more important to him to remain committed to the conversation, even at the cost of death. It is tempting to read *The Apology* or *Phaedo* in the light of the Christian Gospels, and the whole Neoplatonic project of early Christian thought; that is, it is tempting to think that Socrates was merely aimed at dying a martyr's death, sacrificing himself for the sake of a much larger message or agenda. It may even be further tempting to think that Socrates died making the wiser calculation; weighing the death of a martyr against the potential retirement and demise of an old man—eccentric at best and senile at worst.

But while these interpretations may be useful toward reinforcing a variety of contemporary cultural agendas, they do not capture the essence of Socrates's commitment. Socrates had lived out his days as an Athenian citizen. That was his community. He fought in the wars for Athens and labored to reform and awaken its citizenry. If at some point Socrates's beloved city decided that it could not abide Socrates, then that was a decision Socrates would accept out of his own integrity. It was Socrates who chose to live in Athens—and if the penalty for being Socrates (in Athens) was death, then that was his choice. That was the condition of Socrates's union with Athenian dialogue: till death do us part.

Deeply connected to this eternal commitment to dialogue is an absolutely unapologetic responsibility. Socrates is going to be himself at all times. When he wants to pray, he prays. This is not to encourage a selfish or careless approach to prayer for today's pastoral caregiver, but the kind of accompanying confidence here is completely unrecognizable in the state of political correctness. This ownership of self is foundational for more complicated aspects of midwifery. It is impossible to create space through negation if the self is disowned in the first place.

Medicine and Dialogue

The Decalogue about Dialogue

There are some principles that we can derive from dialogue that help inform the midwifery relationship. Some of these principles give us a sense of how to structure dialogues, while other principles suggest why Dialogue is central to spiritual midwifery.

(1) Both parties do not (and cannot) have the same experience of the dialogue.

Sometimes people bristle at the idea of midwifery because its theory includes, but is not limited to, applied techniques and approaches that are not immediately transparent to all participants in the conversation. So maybe this comes across as trickery. There may be deliberate employment of indirect communication. Maybe that looks like outright deception. For many people of faith, coupling Jesus with trickery and deception is just plain unacceptable.

Much of the objection may come from our experiences of how our own trust relationships are formed. Simply, we are forced to form them before we can have any understanding of what we are doing, or even what a relationship is. We have parents that we trust implicitly, well before we can articulate "relationship skills." We are forced to grow in relationships before we understand them, and maybe conclude that understanding and authenticity cannot coexist.

For example, a lot of times we experience intimacy through identical experiences of the same event. This can be true on a micro level (growing up as siblings) or a macro level (thousands of people at a sporting event, or millions of people watching TV). But there are a lot of cases where this expectation is problematic at best and pathological at worst. If we identify the onset of intimacy as a parallel experience, we are vulnerable to psychological fusion, transference, and worst of all, countertransference.

To be sure, there are shared experiences that are sweeter because they are shared, like falling in love with each other. But it is no less sure that limiting the definition of intimacy to having exactly the same experience of exactly the same event is a good way of predisposing a spiritual caregiver to think they are in love.

The real-world implications of these dialogical expectations are simply untenable. It is impossible for a skilled clinician to walk into a patient's room and have the same experience of that event as the patient. The one may be sick, and the other may not be. One may be going through the motions of a very busy day, and the other may be going home. One may be dying sooner, and the other later. Yes, it is the same conversation, but the two parties occupy complementary positions.

(2) Both parties are changed by the dialogue—even as the dialogue unfolds.

This might seem a little contradictory at first. Yes, it is strongly maintained that both parties are not experiencing the same event in the same way, but that does not mean that there cannot be risk on both sides, or that they will not both be changed by the encounter. This is the impact that is felt long after the dialogue is over.

But there's more to it. You can expect to walk away from dialogue having been changed. But this also happens in the present moment. This is the dynamic nature of dialogue. There are two parties involved in the dialogue, and each person has an experience of the other. But they also have an anticipated experience of the mirror reflection from the other person. And that interplay can change things. People change their minds, and they also disguise their minds for a variety of reasons. They are afraid to tell the truth, and often give us exactly what we want to hear. Honesty has to be earned, not assumed. And it can happen in the twinkling of an eye; something in the conversation just clicks and suddenly the person decides to say something they have never uttered before—to anyone.

The dialogue is fundamentally dynamic. Facilitating the dialogue requires the acceptance of the reality that both dialogical parties are changing and relationships are constantly in flux.

(3) People occupy particular and exclusive locations in dialogue (there is responsibility).

Everybody is particular. While there is an egalitarian spirit about the dialogue and people are free to participate as they see fit, it is undeniable that people find themselves in the dialogue uniquely.

Some of this speaks to cultural diversity. We all come from somewhere. We all have a cultural heritage. We all are gendered. We all have a perspective that is informed by our whole being. And it is important to anticipate how our given uniqueness is going to mesh and interweave with the uniqueness of another. And both parity and disparity are significant here. There may be a significant barrier or collision of differences that complicates the midwifery relationship (although it cannot be said too often that many times it is exactly through the paradoxical adaptation of these complications where the midwifery occurs). Likewise, extreme parity and similarity can complicate a midwifery dynamic. Extreme similarity enhances the potential for misunderstanding and overidentification. And the midwife is sensitive to all of this.

But this is more than cultural diversity—there is more to this than accepting that everybody is different and that every relationship is different. Some of the different positions in the dialogue are situationally different and complementary. The one going through the crisis is categorically not in the same position as the person who is sent to help. They are both there for the crisis, but they each hold a very different piece of it.

Many relationships between people are exclusive in nature, that is, they prevent the possibility of other kinds of relationships. This is also true for the spiritual midwife. This is true for many professions (physician, priest, psychotherapist) but we also encounter this in everyday life (parent, sibling, spouse). To fuse these kinds of relationships is a short trip to problems. Any experienced counselor or therapist knows not to counsel their own family. People may want the midwife to step away from the role, and as free persons, such a desire can seem legitimate under the value of autonomy. While midwifery values autonomy, it values context even more highly. The fact is, in midwifery there is always asymmetrical equality.

(4) Dialogues must be created and initiated; they are a mutual act of trust, a microcosmic leap of faith.

Dialogues do not simply "happen." Or, simply, they happen in a very careful way. They are not the result of random, haphazard clumsiness. Consciously or unconsciously, they are the direct result of two parties trying very hard to build something.[3] It takes a lot of effort to create a truly open dialogue. And while effort is required, effort alone may not be enough. Skill and theory can help. These relationships are also a mutual act of trust. But it doesn't end there. They are also a mutual act of hope. And a mutual act of vulnerability.

(5) They have an end and no end.

Spiritual midwives should be cognizant that they have the ability and the authority and the responsibility to decide when the dialogue is over.

At the same time, midwives should also realize that conversation threads are ongoing even after the dialogue is "over." People wonder about things. Seeds are planted; everything doesn't have to be said in one

---

3. Is this really true? I think so. In any dialogue there is a very active interpenetration of the conscious and the unconscious. No, all dialogical partners do not see themselves as "trying really hard to build something," but that doesn't really matter. When a conversation touches on the sacred, it is impossible to conclude that it was all a matter of accident.

interaction. Midwives are responsible for the parameters of the interaction. As stated, they decide when to begin and end an interaction. At the same time, they should seek to gain facility over the empty spaces in the conversation.

There is an abundance of empty space that permeates every dialogue. Yes, there are silences, but there are also distances between interactions. And there are always interruptions. All of these spaces are potential tools of the midwife, and tools the midwife needs to command. This even extends to the empty space that follows a relationship. This is true every time the midwife helps someone take the first step of a transformational journey. There is so much more that the midwife will not get to see or share in.

For emphasis, there are virtually no limits to the midwife's usage of empty space in the dialogue. The midwife can even affect a relationship *before* the dialogue has begun (say, through prayer). And through prayer, a midwife can impact a conversation *even after* it has occurred. Now, obviously, this is not the primary modality of the midwife (that is, to pray for things in future or past tenses), because that is the primary modality of a monastic, not a midwife. But the point is to challenge norms and expectations around time, space, and most of all, empty spaces.

(6) Dialogues are neither aimless nor aimed.

The midwife won't enter into the dialogue with an agenda. Whatever agenda arises must be coauthored. But at the same time, expect the midwife to exercise purposeful movement. Indeed, there is no room for wasted movement. So, the midwife makes discreet assessments and specific interventions, but this is not some kind of predetermined agenda.

(7) Dialogues are marked by mutual consent and mutual assessment.

This is where the equality of dialogue comes in. Although each participant in the dialogue is situated in a particular position (and invariably there will be an imbalance of power here), there remains, nonetheless, a fundamental equality between the partners. The equality is expressed by mutual consent and mutual assessment.

The mutual consent upon which dialogue is predicated is found in a healthy respect for autonomy and vigilance over appropriate boundaries—two sides of the same coin. People have the right to their choices.

The mutual assessment is the simultaneous establishment of trust. It is a dynamic process with changing quantities and entities, and often looks complementary. The ability of the midwife to affect a trustworthy disposition can easily impact the quality of spiritual assessment. Both parties have to decide if the conditions are right for serious labor.

Medicine and Dialogue

(8) Dialogues are relational experiments where other relationships are explored. In the course of dialogue, the Other is invited to explore relationships to various things in his or her life.

Dialogues are typically short-term relationships. In the context of that short-term relationship, the midwife may be invited to share some of that person's most significant relationships and attachments. By connecting to the midwife, a person may have the opportunity to revisit material that was especially formative, or to reframe relationships that are frustrating and painful.

We have feelings about our experiences. These feelings can be understood as relationships. I have a relationship to my health issues, and what they have meant to me over the years. I have a relationship to my prognosis and what my future possibilities are. I can explore these relationships within dialogue, which is, itself, a relationship.

(9) Dialogues are expressed in relational language (rhetoric).

In some ways, this principle illuminates its antecedent. Through relationship between two persons, it is possible to explore many other sacred relationships and attachments. Through trusting the midwife, persons may get to explore some of their most important connections to the world: their faith, their loved ones, even their own personal history.

One of the reasons why the dialogue is so effective at getting to the heart of the sacred relationships is because the very medium of dialogue—language—is itself relational (*n.b.* that "language" is derived from Logos). It is through the exact relationship of grammar that words take on their meaning and exude a life that transcends what is written. Through juxtaposition and contextual conjugation our words find themselves relating to one another and it is only in the relation of these words that we are able to name and share the experiences of the soul. This is what Socrates is getting at with Phaedrus. Language is close to the soul, and this is why midwives work in words—not in the static homily, but in the dynamic dialogue.

It is worth underscoring the truth that silence is a part of language, in both the medium and the mode.

(10) Understanding the relational essence of dialogue, there are many basic and powerful ways to shape the troublesome relationship.

Relationships are at the core of midwifery. In the dynamics of spiritual life, it is not uncommon to find a problematic relationship that is not quickly solved. Maybe it's a relationship with another person, or maybe it's something like a personality trait that is hard to accept. But in most cases, a difficult relationship emerges where it is hard to move forward in life with a sense of freedom. Much of the content of spiritual midwifery deals with some kind of difficult relationship.

Going forward, midwifery offers many ways to affect that relationship. Perhaps it's through a direct aspect of the midwife relationship. Or maybe in fleshing out the language around the problem, there is a way to shift and reframe the grammar of how the problem is experienced.

This deserves some emphasis: there's a lot that spiritual midwifery doesn't have the power to do. If somebody has lost a leg, spiritual midwifery is not going to regenerate any limbs. However, what matters very much is how that person feels about that lost leg; that is, what is the relationship of this person to their loss? And that is very important, because when it comes to all kinds of relationships, spiritual midwifery is very effective. And perhaps this might be the most important thing of all. We all live in a world where loss and limitation are a part of the natural order. In many cases, our relationships to those losses and limitations are more important than the losses themselves. The losses and limitations are merely facts, but the relationships to those facts are where the meaning comes in. And that's exactly where spiritual midwifery has traction.

In sum:

1. Both parties do not (and cannot) have the same experience of the dialogue.
2. Both parties are changed by the dialogue—even as the dialogue unfolds.
3. People occupy particular and exclusive locations in dialogue (there is responsibility).
4. Dialogues must be created and initiated; they are a mutual act of trust, a microcosmic leap of faith.
5. They have an end and no end.
6. Dialogues are neither aimless nor aimed.
7. Dialogues are marked by mutual consent and mutual assessment.
8. Dialogues are relational experiments where other relationships are explored. In the course of Dialogue, the Other is invited to explore relationships in their lives.
9. Dialogues are expressed in relational language (rhetoric).
10. Understanding the relational essence of Dialogue, there are many basic and powerful ways to shape the troublesome relationship.

Part II

Physique and Physics

NAMES ARE TRICKY. GETTING them right is everything; I have often thought that Adam's intended vocation was poetry. It would not have been misleading to title this section "Anatomy and Kinesthetics." When we talk about physique, we are talking about the anatomy of midwifery. The study of anatomy has a classical feel, from the Roman statue to the Renaissance's Vitruvian Man. There is a majesty in this material, as inspiring as the Roman column or the Gothic cathedral. These bones are hallowed.

At the very same time, a sober tone can sound, because anatomy tends to be cadaverous. You can dissect something so much that it feels dead. Aesthetically, this can be a problem for our project because so much of our imagery is bound up in new life. The dangers are clear: we just might kill the thing we are trying to talk about.

Of course, a literal midwife ought to be very familiar with anatomy. Not just its common forms, and not just its variations in presentation, but even significant exposure to its abnormalities. I want to go into some of the detail. We have a metaphor that is robust and a nuanced perspective that can be a useful guide in the care of souls. But there's more, there's an idea resting behind this poetry—a math, a science—that can inform our work. We have a metaphor that has some sufficiency—but there's so much more.

A certain kind of imagination has to precede some of the counterintuitive principles ahead of us. There are certain questions for which only the midwife has the patience to wait. These theories are almost called into being by the perspective of the midwife. You'd have to be comfortable with

Part II—Physique and Physics

working indirectly to even want to integrate this kind of theory into practice. You might be able to enjoy the metaphor of midwifery without much interest in the underlying anatomy, but really grasping the anatomy is only possible for those who have embraced the perspective. And for some, that's all the more compelling.

Chapter 4

The How and the What

> If I speak in the tongues of men and of angels,
> but have not love,
> I am only a resounding gong
> or a clanging cymbal.
>
> 1 CORINTHIANS 13:1

WHAT WE ARE TALKING about is indirect communication. At first thought, the need to talk about "indirect communication" doesn't sound very promising. At best, it sounds unnecessarily technical, and at worst it sounds unnecessarily dishonest. If spiritual things and ideas are to be communicated, why not communicate them as openly and transparently as possible?

Unfortunately, the deepest things cannot be communicated this way. What counselor does his best work by simply telling people what they must do to change their lives? If that were the essence of the therapeutic process, one wouldn't need much more than a diagnosis. But anyone who has ever had anything to do with the therapeutic endeavor—either the counselor or the counselee—knows that just telling people what's wrong with them does not help them.

This is equally true of spiritual work. Telling people that they need God is hardly news. And if people have developed problems in their relationship with God, this "news" is not helpful at all when in comes to fixing the problem. If a pastor stands up in the pulpit and says, "Here is the ultimate

Part II—Physique and Physics

problem," and then follows that with, "Here is the ultimate answer," there is not going to be much more to say. And if the people have been fed, it will not be likely that they have been fed very fully. If they are honest about the sermon, they will find it prescriptive and preachy.

And as obvious as all this is, most people want a little more convincing before they embrace the idea of indirect communication. So, here are some examples that are ordinary in professional spiritual care. Even something as ordinary as offering prayer can be tricky for a chaplain. Lots of chaplains offer prayer all the time, without any appearance of problems or tricks. While prayer can often be a part of a visit, do we really know why the patient or client has consented to pray? Is the patient really free to decline the prayer? If a nice person has come in and listened to an earful of problems, and then wants to pray, is the patient going to say, "No, please don't pray"? They might, but such honesty is rare and ought to be treasured. In order to say no, the person has to risk the newly formed relationship. They must risk the silent judgment of the religious figure in the room.

This dynamic may invoke a spiritual attitude that is antithetical to prayer. If the patient is submitting to prayer only to please or pacify the spiritual caregiver, then this person's deepest longing may not be for communication with God. That's not the worst possible thing—people pray for all kinds of reasons and most of them are probably not ideal (people express all kinds of desires and frustrations to God that have nothing to do with relationship). But it is problematic for the spiritual caregiver to either be unaware of, or choose to ignore, that kind of dynamic. Plenty of clergy recognize the tendency for others to consent to prayer, but they choose to ignore the dynamic and continue the practice because they don't know what else to do. "Yes," they may concede, "this person may be allowing me to pray for all the wrong reasons, but if I can't trust the person to be completely honest with me, I don't know how to do my job." That may not be good enough. Not knowing what else to do is like reading Scripture literally under the argument that God would not allow us to misunderstand divine revelation. One of God's most impressive acts of courage seems to be the relentless determination to be in relationship with us even though we so often misunderstand.

The dynamic involved echoes strongly of the Heisenberg uncertainty principle. In trying to determine the behavior of the utterly small quantum particles, researchers learned that they could not ascertain the speed of a particle without affecting its direction, and they could not ascertain the direction without affecting the speed. The observer could not observe without affecting the particles. And there is a very similar process between clergy and the lay, chaplains and their patients, and spiritual caregivers and their clients. The very attempt to ascertain the desire of the other to pray is quite likely to affect the response given. It is unlikely and unrealistic to think the relationship between persons will have absolutely no impact on what is communicated between them.

The difficulties that are analogous to Heisenberg are not limited to relationships between two. It can be just as hard for one person to identify his or her own spiritual needs. That can be surprising at first; presumably people who are hungry know that they are hungry and even what they hunger for. But the spiritual hunger is different. It is very hard to be engrossed in a given experience and to reflect on that experience at the same time. For a very similar reason, some people say they have a hard time thinking and feeling at the same time (and of course, we are most likely to notice the difficulty when we are trying to think while swept away by very powerful feelings). When we are asked to engage our spirituality, by definition that is very engrossing, and it is very hard to offer immediate reflection of any depth.

Kierkegaard, Objectivity, and Subjectivity

On this point Kierkegaard is unflinching: religion, even in the most general sense, is not a philosophy. That is to say, Kierkegaard's great idea about religion is that it's not an idea at all. What is religion, then? If Kierkegaard were to directly tell us then we'd get the wrong idea; namely, that religion is an idea that can be discussed and communicated like any other.

Objectivity

In secular culture, we have a lot of respect for "objective facts." In the pantheon of facts that dominate our values, objective facts reign supreme. We look to data, research, and studies for guidance. We trust those facts so completely that we could say secular culture places a high value on objective facts.

But Kierkegaard takes the opposite tack. He suggests that objective facts have a low value. Why? Because he wants us to look at objectivity in terms of relationship. If we think about objectivity relationally we can ask, what is the proper role of objectivity in relationship? Rather than using objectivity to inform me about the nature of the object (say, trying to be objective about the nature of a performance), objectivity really informs me about my relationship to the object. I can be objective about a rock that I pass on the street. And as relationships go, the rock is not very important to me.

Disinterestedness is a fundamental aspect of objectivity. I can tell you, objectively, that Edison invented the light bulb, but the fact itself will not change your life. Facts are objective. Nobody really cares when the wheel was invented despite the fact that we all use it. "Objectively understood, there are more than enough results everywhere, but no decisive result anywhere."[1] People can all too easily become passionless factmongers. Kierkegaard acknowledges, "Under the pretext of objectivity the aim has been to sacrifice individualities entirely."[2] So the problems of objectivity are "first, that of not living seriously within the concepts entertained, and, second, forgetting that one is an existing human being."[3]

In forgetting that one is an existing human being, the objective and abstract thinker has become so distanced from life itself that these high-minded ideas clash with reality. The abstract thinker becomes extracted out of life itself. At some point these lofty thoughts have to come back to earth. The effect is like scheduling multiple lunch appointments on the same day, except that the casualty isn't lunch but one's entire existence. It is a duplicitous mistake of trying to follow to mutually exclusive life paths. The result is spiritual madness. As Kierkegaard says, "Spiritually speaking a man's thoughts must inhabit the house in which he lives—or else there is something wrong."[4]

Religion and spirituality necessarily conflict with objectivity—that is, objectivity in the sense of approaching life at arm's length, where by definition spirituality is the thing that matters most to us. Some people try to relate to the religious objectively; for example, someone finds her strength

1. Kierkegaard, *Concluding Unscientific Postscript*, 34.
2. Kierkegaard, *Diary*, 101–2.
3. Gouwens, *Kierkegaard as Religious Thinker*, 32.
4. Kierkegaard, *Diary*, 90.

The How and the What

from the fact that the Bible has been written. Kierkegaard would argue that objectively, this person could never know exactly the facts of how it was written. The "how it was written" is not the historical textual criticism—no, the how is, how do you write a love letter? Once a person relates to the Bible that way the fundamental relationship has changed; "The speculative thinker looks at Christianity as a historical phenomenon."[5] Much of Kierkegaard's ministry is a deliberate attempt to set out to rescue the speculative thinker.

Subjectivity

For the objective thinker, ultimate faith is placed in facts and figures. If only he might know enough, objectively observe enough, then he might be okay. So the objective thinker centers his or her day around the gathering of facts, much like the trading of information around the corporate water cooler. When the thinker finally discovers that the facts are in themselves worthless, a revelation occurs. There is another way of knowing; there is subjectivity.

> Whereas objective thinking invests everything in the result and assists all humankind to cheat by copying and reeling off the results and answers, subjective thinking invests everything in the process of becoming and omits the result, partly because this belongs to him, since he possesses the way, partly because he as existing is continually in the process of becoming, as is every human being who has not permitted himself to be tricked into becoming objective, into inhumanly becoming speculative thought.[6]

The key distinction between objective and subjective thought is simply this: "*Objectively the emphasis is on what is said; subjectively, the emphasis is on how it is said.*"[7]

We tend to think of subjective opinion as that which is inferior to objective truth. But the subjective is that which actually matters to a person. The subjective comes before the predicated reality of the objective.

In other words, Kierkegaard argues that objectivity relates to the relative (things that just happen to occur) as though they were the absolute (things

---

5. Kierkegaard, *Concluding Unscientific Postscript*, 53.
6. Ibid., 73.
7. Ibid., 202 (emphasis added).

Part II—Physique and Physics

that happen for only the most serious, eternal reasons). Subjectivity relates relatively to the relative, and absolutely to the absolute. He argues further,

> If the absolute *telos* does not absolutely transform the individual's existence by relating to it, then the individual does not relate himself with existential pathos but with esthetic pathos—for example, by having a correct idea, but, please note, by which he is outside himself in the ideality of possibility with the correctness of the idea; he is not in himself in existence with the correctness of the idea in the ideality of actuality, is not himself transformed into the actuality of the idea.[8]

Christianity is one of several types of subjective thinking whose scope is aimed at character transformation. Kierkegaard adds, "The Socratic secret—which, unless Christianity is to be an infinite retrogression, can be infinitized in Christianity only by an even deeper inwardness—is that the movement is inward, that the truth is the subject's transformation within himself."[9]

For Kierkegaard, the "how" is ultimately more important than the "what."

All of this is to say that the "The *how* of the truth is precisely the truth."[10] He demonstrates the priority of the "how" in the example of love. "There is no word in human language, not one single one, not the most sacred one, about which we are able to say: If a person uses this word, it is unconditionally demonstrated that there is love in that person."[11] His point is that if there were such a word then it would be the "what." All someone would have to do is speak this "what" and then it would be clear that love lived in that person. But there is no such "what" in matters of love, there is only the "how"—only the ardor of the young man's striving courtship, only the blush on the young woman's cheeks, and only the "how" in matters of truth.

The potential tragedy of religion is that you can get all of the facts right and all of the relationships wrong. Because true spirituality is ultimately subjective, it cannot be bequeathed like a fact. Homiletician Fred Craddock concludes, "It follows that one cannot, therefore, acquire knowledge from a

---

8. Ibid., 387.
9. Ibid., 38.
10. Ibid., 323.
11. Kierkegaard, *Works of Love*, 13.

teacher. Socrates saw his task to be one of helping to remove the hindrances of misunderstanding in order to awaken and evoke truth within."[12]

One of the best ways to get the relationships wrong is to reduce the Almighty to the significance of a single idea. To treat God as though God were a theory, as relativity itself is a theory, is to not understand or know God at all. This is the key message in the work of Jewish theologian Martin Buber. In his groundbreaking work, *I and Thou*, he reminds us that God's primary role in our lives is to not be someone to be talked about, not even as the highest Idea in the world of ideas, but someone that we should be talking to.

Indirect Communication and Midwifery

Going about trying to do spiritual midwifery by only the method of direct communication is a bit like thinking the spiritual task can be solved as easily as, "Burger and fries, please." That's not going to work.

So many times in pastoral care, we hunger for the certainty that is implicit in an objective transaction. This is especially true in the more clinical settings where pastoral care is practiced as a discipline. We yearn for the request that is as literal and comprehensible as ordering fast food through a drive-through. But the spiritual nature of everything we are trying to do defies that kind of transaction.

We see just how complicated the interplay of relationships and the movement of the soul is. Spiritual midwifery is much more than uncovering incorrect ideas about the spiritual life and then replacing them with correct ideas. Indeed, we see that our attitudes and relationships toward those ideas is centrally more important than those ideas themselves—and this is a good thing when we are relating to the Almighty, because the finite can never comprehend the Infinite. Spiritual midwifery is sensitive to both the "how" and the "what"—and it stands at the ready to recognize significant disconnects between the two.

The underlying relationship toward the goal of faith is more important than it is consciously understood. We can think all kinds of things about our tradition. We can have ideas about how the tradition is formed and what it is supposed to mean. But we can work with all of those ideas in a way that never touches relationship. What's more, we see how these subtle relationships can be adversely impacted by attempts at direct communication.

12. Craddock, *Overhearing the Gospel*, 90.

Being too straightforward can obscure the spiritual and sublime from view. We can wind up talking about ideas that have nothing to do with who we really are. If we are not really talking about the core relationships that define us, then we are not going to be able to effect a deeper transformation.

Kierkegaard's Dash[13]

If I say, "This person is standing by himself through my help" ... What am I saying by this? I am saying, "He stands simply and solely through my help"—but then, of course, he is not standing by himself, then he has indeed not become his own master; then, after all, it is to my help that he owes all this—and he is aware of it.

To help a human being in that way is really to deceive him. Yet this is the way in which the greatest beneficence is most often done in this world—that is, in the way in which it cannot be done. Yet this is the way that is especially appreciated in the world....

Many authors use the dash on every occasion of thought-failure; there are also authors who use the dash with insight and taste; but a dash has never truly been used more significantly and never can be used more significantly than in this little sentence—if used, note well, by someone who has accomplished it, if there is such a person—because in this little sentence infinity's thought is contained in a most ingenious way, and the greatest contradiction is surmounted. He is standing by himself—that is the highest; he is standing by himself—more you do not see.... No, from the eyes of the independent one (for if he knows that he has been helped, then in the deepest sense he of course is not the independent one who helps and has helped himself); it is behind the dash.

---

13. Kierkegaard, *Works of Love*, 275.

Chapter 5

The Pangs of Socratic Irony

> The more Socrates tunneled under existence,
> the more deeply and inevitably each single remark had to gravitate
> toward an ironic totality,
> a spiritual condition
> that was infinitely bottomless,
> invisible, and indivisible.
>
> KIERKEGAARD

Socratic irony is the *primus motor* for spiritual midwifery. And if irony is the motor, it is Kierkegaard who provides the physics behind this spiritual engine. *The Concept of Irony* was his master's thesis, the equivalent of our doctoral degree.

But this is not easy going. However much irony meant to Kierkegaard, something as abstract and counterintuitive as irony may not mean that much to the reader. If I'm going to ask for some attention in this treacherous area, the question may fairly arise: is this trip really necessary? Can't we embrace the living metaphor of the midwife without this technical rhetoric?

Well, yes. But irony is extremely important to the underlying mechanics of what this spiritual midwifery is all about.

The reader may counter: fair enough, but shouldn't the spiritual caregiver be more attentive to the divine—more attuned to God—than to some philosophy about irony?

Irony may not be very important to God. But irony is very important to people. This is especially true if Socrates was right when he said, "Rhetoric is like medicine." People's lives are storied. They are constantly telling a story about where they have come from and where they are going. And they work hard on that story, they make life changes and life choices because they are extremely invested in how that narrative holds together.

What's more, one's very personality—one's very self-construct—is also a story. There is a narrative thread that runs through the fiber of our being, and this is exactly why Socrates says that understanding rhetoric is so essential for understanding the soul.

So each of these threads, that is either the narrative of life story or the personality itself, may become knotted. That happens accidently and on purpose. And these two threads can become tangled and knotted together. And this is why irony is so important; it's the basic theory for understanding knots and the human narrative.

Relationships of every kind can take on a narrative, and this is certainly true for the divine relationship. So that one more reason why looking at irony is all that much more important to bring into this dialogue.

Kierkegaard's Irony

Kierkegaard's irony is not really irony as we know it. Normally we think of irony as funny, maybe even a type of sarcastic or cynical humor. Maybe a certain wry attitude. Or we might think of it as a kind of divine torture where the events of the universe align and conspire against the hopes of mice and men. But all of this is off the mark. Completely.

It is better to describe irony as a metaphor gone out of control, as a mischievous child playing with trains. Vehicle and tenor collide in a paradoxical way, except that everything is in control and everything has purposely been set on a collision course, and it is precisely this control and this intention that defines irony.

Some of this echoes with the aforementioned need for indirect communication and remembering back to our conversation about the how and the what. One of the key concepts with indirect communication is that objective language is not suitable for communicating a message that is

The Pangs of Socratic Irony

fundamentally subjective. The "how" is absolutely essential to the "what." What Kierkegaard is drawing on here is the tension between form and content. There is a pristine idea, yes, but then there is the methodology of how that idea is to be communicated. Kierkegaard says that there needs to be a basic congruence between form and content.

This is the hot spark that illuminates his work on irony. Kierkegaard reveals that irony is basically a consciousness of the discrepancy between the inner life (our own interpretation of our experience) and the outer life (what is visible about us to anyone in the world). Again, Kierkegaard is asking us to think about the relationship between form and content. This is not irony in a cynical or comical sense—as though the inner voice is aloof, laughing at all of the shenanigans going on in the outer world. For Kierkegaard irony was not smug sarcasm. Rather it was the deliberate distinction between what is lived and what is communicated, with the direct intent that the communication affects the life and vice versa. That is, the disparity itself between the inner and outer life becomes a significant part of life, and if used correctly it can be a source of tremendous creativity.

Even though Kierkegaard's understanding is much richer than mere figures of speech, literary irony can help bring the whole thing into focus. There is another figure of speech that is erroneously often thought to be ironic. The oxymoron, which two words are paired that at first glance appear completely incompatible, like "bitter" and "sweet." What actually makes the oxymoron is not the intensity of the contradiction but the way in which the terms work together and depend on each other to create a precisely nuanced meaning (i.e., chocolate really is bittersweet). The terms work together additively.

With irony, the two elements of the contradiction are negated and space is created for something new. We usually think of irony when something is being said that either opposes what is actually being communicated or what is actually happening. The greater the distinction, the greater the irony. Artistically, irony is a purposeful and meaningful distinction between form and content where the two are sent into paradoxical juxtaposition. Let's look at narrative irony—*Romeo and Juliet* is a good example. In the final scene, Romeo laments the death of the Juliet even though she is not really dead. The dramatic irony is greatest when both characters wind up dead and eternally separated. Why? Because the whole plan was to feign death as a means of being together. But so far we haven't seen any kind of creative power in irony, only a kind of painful, poetic pathos.

Collision, Contradiction, and Syntax Error

A computer program is a series of logical statements that provide instruction. If the individual instructions make sense the program will run. But sometimes the instructions can create a paradoxical situation. The program might issue a command where the entire content of a disk is erased—including the program that issued the instruction. The logic has turned in on itself and collided with itself in a paradoxical way. The effect is kind of like the "grandfather paradox" in time-travel theory. What happens if you go back in time and kill your grandfather? Would you be born? And if you weren't born, then how would your grandfather die? This sort of quandary is a favorite of philosophers and armchair astrophysicists, but when this kind of thing happens with computers they just crash and stop working.

But something totally different happens with people: they become free. We box ourselves in with these rhetorical statements that shape our lives like a computer program. In Kierkegaard's words, "The ironic figure of speech cancels itself; it is like a riddle to which one at the same time has the solution."[1] At first it seems like he is just talking about lying. But as we will examine later, this is precisely how Jesus uses the parables.

Irony is much more potent when the elements sent into collision are not what is said and the actuality of the speaker, but the inward faith and the outward life. Kierkegaard's thoughtful attention to Socrates illuminates this kind of lived-out irony. Lived-out irony is a dimension beyond verbal irony. In verbal irony, as Kierkegaard says, the speech cancels itself out and we have a linguistic paradox. In lived-out irony, what is canceled out is life itself—life is inverted and we begin to see ironic nothingness.

Visualizing ironic nothingness is difficult at first. If you encounter verbal irony, you feel like your words are being used against you. With lived-out irony, your own existence becomes the convicting evidence against you.

It is the effect of being on the receiving end of one of Jesus' parables.

Kierkegaard tries to describe it this way, "Ironic infinite elasticity, the secret trap-door through which one suddenly plunges down—not one thousand fathoms . . . but into irony's infinite nothing."[2] The secret

1. Kierkegaard, *The Concept of Irony*, 248.
2. Ibid., 26.

trap-door is the paradox itself. Lived-out irony has a kind of intellectual contradiction, like verbal irony, but it also comes into direct collision with the individual's life. Where life was once nothing but positivity, now it is cast into question and doubt. Negativity is born.

It may be helpful to emphasize the scarcity of this type of creativity. People don't think this way very often. Once a century someone comes along and catches a glimpse of that kind of raw possibility. Socratic irony is to midwifery what Derrida's deconstruction was to the whole movement of postmodernism, essentially its guiding light. Indeed, deconstruction and Socratic irony have much in common.

Kierkegaard continues the explanation of irony, using Socrates's death as an example. Socrates does not know any more about death than the rest of us, but through irony Socrates embraces the nothingness (not of death, but the nothingness of his knowledge of death). In so doing, his entire being is literally negated. Another person might have been afraid of their ignorance about death and decided to recant philosophy. By choosing death Socrates allows his whole life to be a witness for philosophy—his life becomes an ironic communication. Kierkegaard's observations about Socrates show us that in death, we witness his utmost essence.[3] For Kierkegaard Socrates's death was the pinnacle of irony in much the same way that Jesus' death was the pinnacle of God's love—through the self-annihilation.[4]

The Maieutic Method

As Kierkegaard progressed in his thought, his irony developed into a theory of communication. It is an intricate theory, sometimes manifested by direct communication and at other times hidden behind an array of pseudonyms. Kierkegaard's literary machinations tease the reader into a relationship with Christ, and he calls the whole process the "maieutic method" because of the Greek term's connotations of midwifery. It is fair to say that Kierkegaard developed an entire theory of spiritual midwifery, if only for literature. His pioneering in the maieutic makes him a unique dialogical partner. Fred Craddock relates, "As Shakespeare used the fool to provide insight, as Faulkner used the idiot to present the profound, as

---

3. Coincidentally the same can be said of Jesus, but it is not a coincidence in that it can be said for exactly the same reason: this person's particular death was the ultimate embodiment of his life's work.

4. Kierkegaard, *The Concept of Irony*, 197.

Part II—Physique and Physics

the New Testament offers the truth from poor widow, beggar, and child, so SK shaped himself into such contours as would make him a vessel to bear the message."[5] (SK is the pseudonym given Kierkegaard by his Reader, and others who love him.)

The maieutic method is essentially negative. Consider Kierkegaard's discussion of the problem of helping somebody see the truth of Christianity in Christendom. Kierkegaard writes:

> Everything is put in terms of reflection. The communicator is characterized by reflection, therefore he is negative—not one who says that he himself is a Christian in an extraordinary degree, or even lays claim to revelations (all of which answers to immediacy and direct communication); but, on the contrary, one who even affirms that he is not a Christian. That is to say, the communicator stands behind the other man, helping him negatively—for whether he actually succeeds in helping some one is another question."[6]

Growth and progress in the maieutic is a lot like developing film; the process requires a negative. In this passage where Kierkegaard describes reflection he means it in a literal sense. Reflection is not a cognitive recollection but more a sense of mirroring and modeling. And as with most mirrors, we find the mirror to be reversed. Rather than impress someone with our piety we refuse to own the Christian name altogether, not because we are ashamed of it but because we are unworthy of it. In this way the Christian category and our relation to it are preserved. The category is preserved because the other person in the maieutic connection has no reason to confuse the doctrine with our own faults. Our relation is preserved when we always uphold the faith as something above us, something we aspire to, and not as something we have already attained. And remember, this is not Kierkegaard's theology in total but only the small part that discusses the maieutic.

Kierkegaard's suggestion to hide our Christianity invariably makes evangelicals bristle and it is worthy of a second note. Evangelicals might bristle because of the Christian imperative to profess and confess Christ. This profession and confession are well and good in the trials of life but rarely suitable for the situation of midwifery. Saying who we are and what we are about can be very different from the work of helping another.

What faithful critics fail to see is that this kind of spiritual maneuvering and posturing is modeled by Christ. In a comparison of Jesus and

---

5. Craddock, *Overhearing the Gospel*, 54–55.
6. Kierkegaard, *The Point Of View*, 43.

Socrates, philosopher Karl Jaspers writes, "But no Christian could have devised words such as: 'Why callest thou me good? there is none good but one, that is, God.' Those words must really have been spoken by Jesus."[7] We might read Jaspers too quickly and look at that as meaningful textual criticism without really respecting the possibility for self-negation. Ordinarily this would be a useful kind of redaction except that in Jesus' case the absolute point was self-negation. Jaspers even notes the respect that the church fathers had for Socrates, and points out that Theodoret knew that "Socrates' insight into non-knowledge prepares the way for faith."[8] But still, Jaspers misses the point. By negating himself, Jesus is able to bring everyone around him into a midwife's relationship. Perhaps Jesus was silent because he was more concerned about Pilate's soul than whether or not he was executed. If only we nervously chatty pastors had that much concern for our parishioners' souls.

Socratic Irony

The full title of Kierkegaard's dissertation is *The Concept of Irony With Continual Reference to Socrates*. He begins the work by introducing us to Socrates. Diogenes Allen tells us about Socrates: "In obedience to the gods, he accepted the task of making his fellow citizens aware of their ignorance of the proper way for a human being to live, that is of how to find a life truly beneficial, and of helping them to realize that the care of the soul is the most important task."[9]

The philosophic tradition emphasizes two biographers, Xenophon and Plato. The trouble with Xenophon's account is that it is extremely apologetic. Plato's work—which Western philosophy has traditionally held as the expert account on Socrates—is much less apologetic, and for that reason Kierkegaard is more favorable to it. But even so, Kierkegaard insists that Plato's personal purposes obscure the uniqueness of Socrates. Where Kierkegaard objects that Xenophon's work is sorry and apologetic, he says that Plato's emphases are poetic and reveal a Socrates who is very divinized and theologically translated, like the description of Jesus we get in the Gospel of John.

---

7. Jaspers, *Socrates, Buddha, Confucius, Jesus*, 74.
8. Ibid., 18.
9. Allen, *Philosophy for Understanding Theology*, 40.

Part II—Physique and Physics

Kierkegaard dislikes both and advances the less prolific and extensive work of the comic playwright Aristophanes. As a comic writer, Aristophanes faithfully preserved Socrates's tongue-in-cheek for all of history to see, and we might remember that Socrates's contributions to the doctrine of dialogue were no less significant or revolutionary than the contributions to the doctrine of the soul. Psychoanalytic thinker Jaspers agrees, "Conversation, dialogue, is necessary for the truth itself, but now, as the instrument of Socratic philosophizing, it became something different: a conversation that aroused, disturbed, compelled men's innermost souls."[10]

Why did Kierkegaard dislike apologetics? Apologetics is ill-suited for a description of the man who refused to apologize under the threat of civic execution. The basic thrust of Kierkegaard's dislike is that the one who lived and died for the purpose of becoming a gadfly in the ear of his people is no longer a gadfly but through apologetics metamorphosizes into something else, perhaps a ladybug or even a butterfly—something pretty to look at and not worth squashing at all. Kierkegaard says it this way:

> Indeed, Xenophon succeeded in this to such a singular degree that one would be more inclined to believe that it was Xenophon's objective to prove that it was foolishness or an error on the part of the Athenians to condemn Socrates, for Xenophon defends Socrates in such a way that he renders him not only innocent but also altogether innocuous—so much that we wonder greatly about what kind of daimon must have bewitched the Athenians to such a degree that they were able to see more in him than in any other good-natured, garrulous, droll character who does neither good nor evil, does not stand in anyone's way, and is so fervently well-intentioned toward the whole world if only it will listen to his slipshod nonsense.[11]

Kierkegaard mourns the lack of the Socratic barb in Aristophanes. The Socratic barb was a stinging remark or harsh response in the Socratic dialogue that brought the other into direct, tangible contact with irony's "infinite nothing." Kierkegaard clarifies, "With Socrates, rejoinder was not an immediate unity with what had been said, was not a flowing out but a continual flowing back, and what one misses in Xenophon is an ear for the infinitely resonating reverse echoing of the rejoinder in the personality (for

---

10. Jaspers, *Socrates, Buddha, Confucius, Jesus*, 6.
11. Kierkegaard, *The Concept of Irony*, 16.

The Pangs of Socratic Irony

as a rule the rejoinder is straightforward transmission of thought by way of sound)."[12]

There are several useful observations to lift up out of Kierkegaard's distinction. First, we see the juxtaposition of form and content—for Socrates's rejoinder was not in "immediate unity with what had been said." Thus, the form of the Socratic response was not directly congruent with the content of the previous conversation.

Second, even though there is this paradoxical nature of the rejoinder, Kierkegaard still considers it an effective, legitimate, and direct way of linking two people by thought. He uses the word "straightforward."

Third, Kierkegaard beautifully rotates the phrase "*infinitely resonating reverse echoing of rejoinder.*" The spiritual midwife has two ears and one of them has to be infinitely tuned to the other giving birth. But the other ear must be exactly as Kierkegaard says—it must be extremely sensitive to these negatives and ironies if the midwife has any intention of speaking at all.

These ironies are *infinite*, for they stretch all the way from despair to hope, from whatever is lacking to whatever is needed, and from the vastness that separates any one person from another. These ironies *resonate*, for when all has been said—and more importantly, when all has been left unsaid—they will vibrate the entire being of the hearer.

These ironies are *reverse*, because they are paradoxical and necessarily are counterintuitive and flow upstream in the stream of consciousness.

These ironies *echo*, like any truth does, and when the midwife has finished everything that is necessary, it is these ironies that will repeat themselves to the hearer. Paradoxical irony allows the midwife to get through the mess and complexity of ordinary discourse and everyday experience to get to a place that is conducive—in fact, inductive—to bringing forth new life.

Where does this get us? Anticipating and understanding Socratic irony does more than giving us a new tool to express ourselves and get our points across. Really understanding irony can give us a new capacity for hearing what is said.

Irony in the Wild

When Kierkegaard gets on a roll, it is hard to envision how these ideas actually move. He coins a phrase like "infinite nothing," which is at once abstract and poetic. But what does it mean? How do you come into contact

12. Ibid., 18.

Part II—Physique and Physics

with it? One of the chaplaincy interns approached me about a difficult patient interaction. A couple was hoping to have a healthy baby and what had been a completely normal pregnancy ended in sorrow. Apparently the umbilical cord had gotten tangled around the baby's neck.

The intern had offered some very good pastoral care, spending time with the family, helping hold the heavy sadness in the room. The intern resisted the temptation to offer easy answers and hopeful interpretation. There was no silver lining to be found, as none was needed. After the experience the intern found me to discuss a difficulty. "Things went okay with the family," he said, "but the head nurse was very disturbed. She had to excuse herself from the room because she was emotionally devastated."

This is not uncommon, especially on a labor and delivery unit. The trajectory of birth points toward life, and the deaths that do occur can be heartbreaking for all involved. It can be uniquely poignant and ironic for the affected caregivers because of the collision of personal and professional needs. Professionally, there is a need to demonstrate efficacy and it's hard to do that and integrate emotions at the same time. Personally, the death of a baby is gut-wrenching and it threatens to devour every trace of meaning in human life. How can something so horrible actually be happening?

The trainee continued, "The head nurse was really broken up about it, but I don't know how to offer her support." It is a problem. It is very tricky to offer support to hard-core caregivers like doctors and nurses. They see themselves as the dispensers of care, the givers, and they are very resistant to the idea of accepting help. Any attempt to meet that need directly is likely to be met with a brush-off.

What I suggested was that the intern approach the situation by identifying himself as the locus of care. Approach the head nurse, and say something like, "I'm new here, I'm just learning about chaplaincy, and I need some support. How on earth do you cope with tragedies like that?"

So, this is what happened. The head nurse met with the intern and assured him that she didn't need help. But when she saw that he was the one in need of support, she sat down for twenty minutes, and allowed herself to really cry. By understanding what kinds of conflicts would emerge for a head nurse, it became possible to offer her a taste of that "infinite nothing." Once we understand how the ironies are pointed, coming up with approaches to circumvent the resistance is easy. We can either choose to

The Pangs of Socratic Irony

recreate the resistance that binds people, or step around it. But the choice is ours.

In her article "The Midwife, Storyteller, and Reticent Outlaw," Brita Gill-Austern emphasizes that giving voice is part of midwifery. She wants to address "the experience of feeling silenced."[13] But simply approaching the nurse and asking if she would like to talk is not going to give voice; it's giving the opportunity for a polite refusal. Employing irony allows for something else, and gets at the heart of the matter by evoking voice—by "hearing this voice into being."

Another example came up with a mental health support group. This was an acute and diverse population. Many of the patients had dual-diagnoses and this was an inpatient program. This is not a population that has a lot of success with life choices. And that was exactly what I wanted to explore in a workshop.

I started with a little parable. "Imagine if I woke up this morning and I was really tired. Let's say I was tired of going to work every day. Let's say I was going to quit my job and take my last paycheck and buy all the lottery tickets I could. Maybe I was feeling really lucky and really tired of working. Do you think that would be true hope or false hope?"

It seems like an obvious question with an obvious answer. And yes, there is a lot about this question that is obvious. But it is not a question without its own tricks; namely, the people that I was asking are very much the kind of people that struggle with questions like this. These are people who struggle to function in life and they struggle to make good choices. And to pose the question to them directly is to put them in a situation where they well run the risk of making a poor choice again.

That is, until I asked them to advise me. By appreciating the underlying irony of the situation, that they have a hard time with choices like this, and by inserting myself as the object of care, something amazing happened. Suddenly, all those life lessons are no longer courses to be repeated, but can become a curriculum to teach from. Each person, in turn, was able to tell me that it was false hope and why. Appreciating irony allowed me to frame the question in such a way that the patients' basic struggles would not be repeated and recreated, but a different conclusion could be envisioned entirely.

---

13. Gill-Austern, "The Midwife, Storyteller, and Reticent Outlaw," 221.

Part II—Physique and Physics

Irony and the Midwife

Manipulating irony can help others find empowerment around their own life narratives. People become blocked and trapped by life's paradoxes and understanding that can point the way. However, there are also two important considerations about irony and the midwife. These considerations can help the midwife examine her own relationship to irony. First, appreciating irony can help define the work and evaluate it. Am I using this relationship effectively to meet its goals? I know what I'm trying to achieve, but is there a meaningful mismatch between form and content so that I'm working against myself? How does my own personage come into conflict with what I am trying to do? The tension between form and content becomes a useful yardstick.

Awareness of irony also provides an appreciation for the dangers around dual relationships. Dual relationships are those where we relate to the other on more than one level, maybe as friend and counselor, or as colleague and chaplain. The challenge that ensues is that the prophetic voice of the office may conflict very much with the other relationship (be it as friend or family). Irony appreciates that all relationships may not support all dialogues, and therefore helps create a therapeutic sense of caution.

Finally for the midwife, irony offers an excellent framework for understanding some of the more dangerous, painful, and confounding risks in pastoral care. I discovered this when working with some interns around the problem of unwanted sexual attention. This dynamic can emerge with both sexes, but it is more prevalent with female pastoral caregivers and male recipients of care for many reasons. It dawned on me that this is not a harassment issue, this is an irony issue and it's a dynamic that is not limited to sexual themes (although sexual themes can be the most destructive). When an intern is trying to go into a room and minister for God only to have that misconstrued by the patient as something sexual, the result is painful and confusing. It can shake one's sense of religious vocation. But it's not limited to sexual identity, and it can occur along any intimate aspect of personhood, either race, religion, age, physical disability, or sex. When you are rejected or misunderstood at a very basic level of personhood, it can feel like a cosmic condemnation. Understanding the ironic dynamics is the first step to demystifying such a painful and confusing experience, and because the dynamics are properly understood, there is no reason to infuse them with more significance than they require.

In sum:

- Socratic irony is a useful framework for understanding some of the more complicated relationships and dynamics of spiritual midwifery. This science of rhetoric has a rich tradition. There is a clear rationale for the ideas behind midwifery, even if these ideas are paradoxical and hard to communicate.
- These techniques have been used throughout history, both by philosophers and theologians, both in speech and in writing.
- Knowing irony helps us express and understand, to both speak and listen.
- Kierkegaard also shows us how some of these philosophical ideas can point to a spiritual way of being in the world. Jaspers rightly says, "It is a kind of thinking which does not permit man to close himself."[14]
- Socratic irony is a way of using rhetoric and the limits of language to create a verbal experience that will resonate a kind of spiritual experience.
- Appreciating irony is also helpful to the midwife in self-evaluation, boundaries, and processing painful encounters that affect their personhood.

---

14. Jaspers, *Socrates, Buddha, Confucius, Jesus*, 21.

Chapter 6

Seduction, Surrender, and Negation

> But I alone am drifting, not knowing where I am.
> Like a newborn babe before it learns to smile,
> I am alone, without a place to go.
> Others have more than they need, but I alone have nothing.
> I am a fool. Oh, yes! I am confused.
> Others are clear and bright,
> But I alone am dim and weak.
> Others are sharp and clever,
> But I alone am dull and stupid.
> Oh, I drift like the waves of the sea,
> Without direction, like the restless wind.
> Everyone else is busy,
> But I alone am aimless and depressed.
> I am different.
> I am nourished by the great mother.
>
> LAO TZU

NEGATION IS A POWERFUL tool in spiritual midwifery and it is one of the most important postures. It is also one of the most abstract and counterintuitive ideas that needs explication. What if we come across someone who is not experiencing much movement in their spiritual life, and we suspect that this is so because their core relationships are problematic? On the one hand, this is good because midwifery con-

Seduction, Surrender, and Negation

cerns itself with relationship and movement. But on the other hand, it does pose the question: how is the work to be done?

If the midwife comes and says something like, "I think you are experiencing this impasse with God because you are struggling with your past. Perhaps we ought to talk about forgiveness," how exactly do we think that will go? Is it likely that the other person will say, "You are quite right—I have never thought of that, let us talk about forgiveness"?

Probably not. But we can now say why not in the terms that we have just defined. Without meaning to, the would-be midwife has probably just inserted herself between the other person and the very work that they need to do. The credibility of the idea—in this case, trying to do some work in the area of forgiveness—will be a function of the other person's acceptance of the midwife. If the midwife is received as the expert on the subject, and this probably requires that the midwife exudes a spirituality that is convincing to others, then that person may begin to think about what the midwife has had to say, kind of like going to a doctor. If the doctor is recognized as a true physician, we will take his advice.

The problem is that spirituality seldom carries enough of this objective quality for this type of approach to be successful. This is exactly why spirituality is not the ideal topic for objective communication. Spirituality is primarily a subjective phenomenon. But in this instance, the midwife has inserted herself, both her relationship and her trustworthiness as a person, between the other person and spiritual movement. Now, in order to make any progress, the other person has to navigate around the midwife in addition to whatever blockages that they started out with. This is why it is so important that the midwife takes pains not to communicate subjective truths objectively.

It is natural that the careful reader be somewhat perplexed. If we cannot communicate directly, how do we do it? There are lots of ways, and one of the most available is through negation. The difficulty in the above scenario is that the would-be midwife is overinvolved in the communication. An answer to that is to balance the equation by removing oneself. If this hypothetical person could do some work with forgiveness, without getting snared on the personage of the midwife, it might be possible to resume a small measure of spiritual movement. Undoubtedly, other problems would arise in the spiritual life—that's the way of things—but whatever the problem is, it would not be forgiveness.

Part II—Physique and Physics

In this case, the success of the negation depends upon the ability of the midwife to offer forgiveness completely unattached and distinct from the experience of the midwife as a person. That's how it works. Maybe the midwife can help the person by reflecting on someone with a similar story. Maybe the midwife is "reminded" of a similar situation where forgiveness is the obvious way through—but for some reason, it is not so obvious to the midwife. Who knows? Maybe it is the midwife that is in need of forgiveness. The possibilities are endless.

Perhaps, in a chaplaincy setting, the midwife is trying to support a family through a difficult meeting with the hospital staff. In the context of the hospital, where grave and serious things happen all the time, it is all too easy for these meetings to have an antagonistic feel and take on a polarized quality. When people are talking about the illness and possible death of a loved one, emotions are charged and volatile and it is easy to see things in terms of us against them. In that cauldron of intense feeling and complicated decision-making, the last thing both parties need is a complicated personality. Already, the family is likely to view the spiritual caregiver as "one of them." And it's equally plausible that medical staff may have misgivings about bringing someone without any medical expertise into the conversation.

If the midwife can enter into the dialogue—which probably looks more like an involved dance than a typical dialogue—without tangling herself up on either side, there can be a crucial role to play. That role in working with groups probably looks very different from working with individuals. Groups don't always want or need to work on spiritual movement (although, it is true that sometimes they do). But there are plenty of other movements that groups and families need to make. Making a serious life decision in a hospital can be one of those. In today's healthcare, decisions are sought very quickly and there maybe be complicated family dynamics or other family processes that have to be completed before the decision can be made (the family may have to do some grief work, for instance). A midwife will be concerned with dynamic movement—and that is the perfect antidote for people stuck in catch-22s and other entrenched positions.

Whether in working with individuals or groups, negation is a useful tool for the midwife because it helps manage the confusion between direct and indirect communication. Negation can make it possible for the other person to think about the matter at hand—and not to think about the midwife. The metaphor of the midwife and the practice of negation complement each other and each reinforces the other. Negation helps the midwife remember that the midwife is necessarily on the periphery of the central work. And the midwife who understands the work of midwifery is able to bring creativity and ease to the method of negation.

The Ministry of Absence

Within the discipline of pastoral care, so much gets said about the "ministry of presence" that it is nearly impossible to say too much about the ministry of absence—but, yes, since *absence* is the operative term, it is possible to say too much. Doing the topic justice would require a different treatment altogether.

But it is not necessary to say everything to say something. Many times in discussions of pastoral care, "the ministry of presence" is often uttered. The ministry of presence is one of the rich traditions to have emerged from this work with "living human documents." It is a powerful idea. In a nutshell, the idea is that there are many times and places where it is not necessary to do, or especially to say, the right thing. It is enough to be there. And any approach that encourages presence over action, silence over chatter, can't be all bad. Being there is a sufficient challenge in itself. That requires facing a cluster of intense emotions that most people do their best to avoid. It often means embracing acute sadness, grief, and a profound powerlessness.

At its best, the ministry of presence draws deeply from an incarnational theology. Because someone was there, and present, a deeper connection was made. It can seem like such a person is heaven-sent. In the best of the priestly tradition, it can seem like such a person is a representative of God. What's more, there are places where the ministry of presence is the ideal response. There are many situations where people can only focus on the present crisis, and the attempt to direct them anywhere else can only be called inappropriate. When people are waiting for someone to come out of surgery, the best response can often be to wait with them—and quietly.

The ministry of presence runs into problems when it becomes the only tool of the spiritual caregiver, when it becomes the primary modality for doing pastoral care without question. The caregiver can slide the slippery slope into thinking that just showing up is enough, that just attending human beings in crisis transcends all assessment, intervention, and ultimately, accountability. Why do you do what you do? And for some, the ministry of presence is the answer, simply because there is no other answer.

Part II—Physique and Physics

At the end of the day, the ministry of presence still emphasizes what the caregiver is doing: namely, being present. Paradoxically, this phrase that once emphasized what the caregiver doesn't have to do or say, can have the effect of amplifying the opposite impulses. Ministry of presence is a decidedly "glass-half-full" orientation. So much of the pastoral care wisdom that has emerged over the last fifty years has this aphoristic, kerygmatic quality. Phrases get passed on and are trusted with the authority of Scripture. "Ministry of presence" is one of those phrases. Because it has been passed along as a pastoral care truth, and because it is often tested, it is then never questioned. Ever. Its limits and *a priori* assumptions are never examined.

There are other possibilities. If the ministry of presence ultimately underscores the positive functionality of the spiritual caregiver, is there another way—something that reaches out for what the caregiver doesn't do? If we are not concentrating on the presence of the caregiver, maybe we can listen for the presence of the divine. There are all kinds of ways that the presence of the caregiver can create a formidable barrier to the spiritual work that needs to be done. It is hard enough to resist the pressure of making a good impression. It is easy to fall into the narcissism of being accepted or rejected. It is already tempting to begin a relationship and succumb to the seduction of being liked. It is these kinds of distractions that derail spiritual work and turn it into a lesser experience of socializing. A new metaphor is needed to disturb the false peace that has grown around the ministry of presence. A new metaphor can call this colloquialism into question, where it can then be restored as a useful tool—like any other tool, with specific limits and applications.

This is where the ministry of absence comes in. The ministry of absence calls us to look at all the things a spiritual caregiver doesn't do. And in the process, we are encouraged to own a more comprehensive picture of the pastoral relationship—indeed, as the prayer suggests, the things done and the things left undone. We are responsible for all of it, are we not? By the same token, breathing doesn't take us very far if we categorically exclude the possibility of exhaling.

There are specific maneuvers and techniques that facilitate the ministry of absence, but its greatest value is hermeneutic; not simply another set of techniques and approaches, either to do or not to do, as a kind of robotic gimmick of ensuring some kind of standardization of pastoral care. Rather, embracing the ministry of absence restores a trust in the holiness of the interaction between persons created by God. It is a move away from formulas of certainty, and a move toward a creative openness that begins to shape the way the entire relationship is experienced. Instead of aiming for a goal that tends to hope the other person will be better off because of some kind of encounter with us, the ministry of absence hopes that we will go unnoticed. It is not likely to be spiritually transformative if a hospital patient remembers the personal details about a visiting chaplain. But it makes all the difference in the world if the patient doesn't remember a thing about the chaplain, but now views their hospitalization as a way of reconnecting with God. The ministry of absence serves as a constant reminder that the greatest work is not from clergy or caregiver, but God. While the ministry of presence can be corrupted and misunderstood as the business of being liked and customer satisfaction, the ministry of absence forever reminds us that there are larger questions of meaning at work.

The practice of midwifery is about remembering where the work lies. In any birth, it is never the midwife that does the most work. And even the one who is doing the laboring realizes that the new life is a blessing from God.

Socratic Negation

The way of negation is a continual *modus operandi* for Socrates throughout the entire *Dialogues of Plato*. Each dialogue offers an endlessly inventive way for getting oneself out of the way of a true philosophic inquiry. In some cases, Socrates begins the inquiry by finding an expert about something that he needs to learn. In many instances, Socrates is free to admit that he does not know or have the answer. In other cases still, Socrates will argue with himself—to the effect of contradicting pages and pages of philosophic argumentation. Why would he do that? Surely, the great philosopher could spare his dialogical partner (and Plato his reader) pages and pages of philosophic error? But the process—the midwifery—that Socrates is working is a more significant process of transformation than merely spewing some kind of objective idea or theory. Socrates is willing to take more than one left turn and follow more than one rabbit trail for the sake of the soul of his compatriot and fellow citizen.

The entire figure of Socrates is enshrouded in this reputation of negation to an almost-mythic degree. Legend has it that the Oracle at Delphi said that no one in Athens was wiser than Socrates. We can conclude that this is a part of Socrates's PR that he really owned and advertised because

Plato put this in his most historical dialogue—Socrates's actual trial where more than 500 people were present. These details could have been immediately falsified. Socrates could not believe this commendation of the Oracle because he was convinced that he knew nothing. This is the ultimate negation and it takes more than a little courage to weave it into your defense when you are on trial for your life. So, Socrates took it as his vocation to find people who knew more than he did. What he found were a lot of people that erroneously thought they knew more than they did, but Socrates at the core knew he knew nothing. He concluded that, if anything, it was this authentic piece of non-knowledge that made him the wisest of all.

Socrates made his vocation the work of this negation. And it is not surprising that he chose to die in the same way that he lived—by practicing negation. It seems as though Socrates could have accepted exile or escaped, but instead of that faced execution by drinking poison. Facing death in this way means a lot of different things. To some extent, it means that Socrates viewed the task of being an Athenian citizen a solemn responsibility even unto death. But in the context of negation, realizing that suicide is the ultimate negation, Socrates saw that allowing himself to be put to death by the state in this way meant more for his lifelong project of teaching others through negation than the possibility of living longer.

The Theology of Negation

From the earliest beginnings of the Jesus movement, a type of spiritual negation lies very close to the heart of the message. The highest holy days are saturated with it. From the coming of Jesus in the incarnation to his death and resurrection, Jesus's consistent project dealt with negation, usually through different forms of surrender. And just for a moment, it is worth recognizing that the greatest works of Christ—the ones referenced by the eucharistic liturgy as the great mystery of faith: that Christ has died, Christ is risen, Christ will come again—are each marked by passivity and negation. For starters, these are all things that happened to Jesus, and in many cases Jesus did not have the wherewithal to do anything differently. Even when Jesus seems to be the most passive and ineffective, reality-altering events are unfolding. The death of Christ negates the coming of the Christ child and the work of his ministry. The resurrection negates the very death of Jesus—and, in fact, negates the power of death itself.

Seduction, Surrender, and Negation

Paul explores this theology in a near-mystical fashion. In Philippians, he says, "Christ poured himself out, taking the form of a servant" (Phil 2:7). It is this spiritual emptying we find again and again in the words and actions of Jesus. Whether it is the "last that shall be first," the washing of the disciples' feet, or the divestiture of piety by performing miracles on the Sabbath, it is a motion that is recurrent in patterns large and small. These kinds of movements and values are repeatedly expressed in the ministry of Jesus Christ.

Consider the Lord's Supper. Jesus spoke this way often, either in terms of living water, or living bread, but the context here is what is so impressive. This event led to the central ritual of the entire Christian movement. And through the Eucharist, we have superimposed a kind of sense on the Lord's Supper interpreted through later experiences of death and resurrection. Today when we celebrate Communion, the meal resymbolizes the sacrifice of Jesus. But the meal as meal was already a metaphoric and symbolic act. Like the "living water" offered to the woman at the well, Jesus was offering himself as a symbolic food. Although unlike the "living water" that gives life and quenches eternal thirst, with the bread and wine Jesus says that it is clearly himself on the menu. What is important here is recognizing that when Jesus uses a food-based metaphor to describe a spiritual reality—there is already a bit of negation at work in the poetry alone. What is doubly interesting at the Last Supper are the multiple layers of negation. At a meal with the betrayer, Jesus performed a compound negation by describing a spiritual truth with the poetic food image like the living water, but then brings that into a negating collision with his own personhood. "This is my blood, this is my body."

After two thousand years of tradition, we are inclined to shrug off the strangeness. It's an abstract ritual that we don't think about too closely, and if we do we are likely to ignore the inherent strangeness by thinking that rituals of meaning have their own historical evolution—and perhaps its not so strange that Jesus would speak this way to a community that had an active practice of burnt offerings of animal flesh.

But perhaps we should allow ourselves to be shocked by the jarring idiom. Even if the disciples appreciated the reference to the atonement theology of their tradition, it's not exactly a comforting thought. The eerily cannibalistic overtones would have been awkward and strange to anyone. Perhaps the key into this strange statement is not the sacrificial economy of the temple period, but the principle of negation. Of course, when food is consumed, it is annihilated, it's gone. At some level, Jesus is setting up an equation with the bread and wine. By ingesting and incorporating the incarnation, we can have a new kind of life. But before we do anything, that bread and wine are offered freely from Jesus by a process that looks very much like what Paul describes in the "pouring out" of spirit. Negation is the doorway to the entrance of divine mystery. It's hard to appreciate the prerequisite of negation because our attention has skipped over that for two thousand years, fixated on the elements of Communion, and tried to understand our part in the sacrament.

It may be worth adding that where ideas about Christian negation have emerged, the discussion has often been confused. Negation is not the same kind of idea as popular passivity, and it has absolutely nothing to do with the submission of the oppressed. These may be areas where the principles of negation are likely to be misinterpreted. Jesus does not practice a kind of self-hatred because that is what we are supposed to do—and there are some communities where Christianity has been pathologized that way. Perhaps the clearest distinction is that the negation practiced by Jesus is never the point, but always a means to an end—a larger process that usually involves inducing the movement of another.

One of the most frequent places where Jesus practices negation is through the rhetoric of the parables—and we will examine this much more closely later on.

What Does Negation Look Like?

Because negation is not the goal, but rather a means to an end, there is not one prescription for what it looks like, or how to do it. Negation is more of a value or a concept than a specific method or series of steps. There are lots of ways to do it, and the different ways will also range in their impact. But if done right, the impact is never noticed. Even a little self-effacing humor should not stand out and evoke pity.

There are good reasons to incorporate negation into the tool kit of the midwife. Ultimately, the focus of the relationship is not on the midwife, but on the one giving birth. A healthy dose of negation can keep the ego in check, and make sure the attention is directed where it needs to go. Negation is one of the best ways to create a space in relationship for someone else to do spiritual work; perhaps wherever creation is involved it always

Seduction, Surrender, and Negation

happens *ex nihilo*—there always needs to be a creative void if new life is to emerge.

What's more, there are some technical aspects that deal with the problems of direct and indirect communication that can be solved or avoided altogether through negation. There are inherent complications in spiritual midwifery, and there are ways that an overly pronounced personality can undermine the spiritual work.

Negation and the ministry of absence can become a complementary alternative modality to the ministry of presence. The ministry of presence can easily lose sight of the work that God is doing when we are still, because, after all, it is we who are offering the presence. A negative orientation nurtures an inward circumspection. Thinking about negation and the ministry of absence as a basic way of approaching ministry can be a kind of frame or vessel for the pastoral relationship that can guard us from the temptations of being liked and accepted (where the real work is in the birth—not cultivating popularity). Even without a specific context and instance of negation, merely valuing the principal of negation can change the way we approach and form relationships.

I remember one very contentious meeting between a family and the medical staff of the hospital where I was serving at the time. The medical opinions were clear and in consensus: the patient was not going to recover and healing would not come from more treatment. The family had been convinced that along the way, the best course of treatment had not been followed, and there had been other opportunities and possibilities.

This might not seem like an ideal application for negation. This was a real case with real people and it might be inappropriate to offer something so theoretical in the face of such active grief. Both sides were heavily armed with facts, and both parties seemed to think that if they presented the facts hard enough, the other side would have to relent and surrender.

From where I was sitting, it didn't seem like this was about facts at all, but rather, feelings. Moving forward was going to be an emotional exertion, not an intellectual one. For this family to really engage the reality of a gravely ill loved one, they were going to have to feel their way through—whatever decisions they came to. In the context of medicine and science, though, feelings are the liability. They are not trustworthy when compared to facts, and in the family meeting, both parties had ulterior motives for sticking to the facts.

Somehow, feelings were going to have to be brought into the room, and this was exactly the form that the negation took. In this instance, the chaplain needed to become emotion itself—and I needed to embrace all of the stigma of being emotional and irrational. And so I did. I said that I was sorry about everything, and I really tried to connect with the experience of seeing a loved one in that condition. I apologized for things—things I had no control over. I was sorry, and probably a sorry sight.

I also demonstrated that emotions could be engaged and that I could lose face, because in that situation, my saving face was not important. What was important was a family that was very much stymied in their emotional work because they were trying to conform those feelings to the world of facts. And what's more, my colleagues, who were excellent caregivers, were not giving the help that was needed, because they too thought they had to stick to the facts.

As long as that family was going to prop up their anger with their carefully selected facts, they were not going to be able to move through the valley of grief that was clearly before them. Even if they were right about all their facts—which was debatable, and the trick is to avoid the debate—this was a family facing grief. It was the goal of the midwife to lead them to a future where the grief could begin.

Chapter 7

Inductive Logic and Being Induced

> You cannot solve a problem from the
> same consciousness that created it.
> You must learn to see the world anew.
>
> EINSTEIN

Deductive logic is an important concept within the framework of spiritual midwifery, because it is largely the theoretical backdrop that spiritual midwifery stands in direct contrast to. If spiritual midwifery asks us to think differently about the art of the care of souls, how were we thinking in the first place? What do we think about our very thinking?

When most people talk about logic and "being logical," it is largely deductive logic that they are talking about. In the West, the only kind of logic that is widely respected is deductive logic.

These ideas gained their dominance through the work of Aristotle, who really shaped movement and vector of deductive logic through his syllogisms. Perhaps he is to be credited with the genesis of the great scientific impulse that has so completely propelled our civilization to its almost-magical level. If A is greater than B, and B is greater than C, then we can assume that A is greater than C. This is also the transitive property of equality. We can know a set of things about A, and if B is a subset of A such that all of the statements about A also apply to B, and then we see that C is a similar subset of B, then all of the things we can say about A also apply

Part II—Physique and Physics

to C. A famous syllogism reads: All men are mortal, and Socrates is a man; therefore, Socrates is mortal.

The basic pattern of movement is that if we can say something about the general, then the laws that govern the general will also apply to the specific and particular.

The reasoning is sound, but it didn't really become such a dominant way of thinking in the West until the Enlightenment. The Age of Reason following the Enlightenment really pursued deductive reasoning leading to determinism, materialism, and the modernism that captured the West at the turn into the twentieth century. Deductive reasoning fits in very well with determinism, which suggests that the world is governed by very regular laws and principles. If we understand the laws that describe how reality moves, and we understand the exact state of reality at the present moment, then we ought to be able to accurately predict how reality will be in the future. This is determinism in a nutshell. This is also the Newtonian perspective. A more sophisticated determinism concedes that even if it is not possible to examine the exact nature of reality at precisely one moment, the universe is still governed by very rigid rules even if the outcomes are currently unknowable to us.

Deductive reasoning and this kind of ontological determinism that has led to our control over science are very powerful ways of engaging the world. By use of these conceptual tools entire civilizations have been built, and entire civilizations have been destroyed. And it is fair to suggest that ideas with this much raw power appeal to the universal human appetite for control.

It is no coincidence that modern psychology was born somewhere between rationalism and determinism. As we began to understand the physical and chemical forces that shaped the material world, it also seemed evident that the inner world was affected by its own kinds of imposing forces. Now all we had to do was understand them. And much of the thrust behind Freud's project was establishing psychology properly as a science. This is why psych majors today still do experiments with rats and take courses in statistics—that modernist impulse is still there.

To be fair, there have been many thinkers and contributors to the field of psychology that don't view people or life itself through a deterministic lens.

That said, the deterministic history of psychology is very important because the determinism is a conceptual world view at the core of many principles in psychology. Determinism was the foundation upon which the house of academic psychology was built. And what's more, academic psychology has had a considerable influence over the development of the discipline of pastoral care. By temporal proximity alone, today's student or practitioner of pastoral care has a lot more opportunity to understand the mind of psychology, than, say, the mystical spirituality of medieval Christianity. Further, the contemporary mind is better suited to receive the quasiobjective theory passed on through direct communication, than the subjective spirituality that really cannot be communicated directly. Simply, the sublime is harder to get. The direct and the literal translate easier.

Unfortunately, what we end up with is a kind of borrowed authority twice-removed. Whereas early psychology struggled and wrestled to be received by the academy as a credible science, many developments in pastoral care today try to borrow the same kind of authority from psychology.

We live in a world that is still very informed by Newtonian values; we live in a world that expects measurable results in a timely fashion. Any professional pastoral caregiver beyond the church has felt this pinch, and profoundly so (although it is not much of a reprieve if the typical parishioner has the same cultural catechesis). To put it bluntly, the hospital chaplain serves in a world driven by results and is forced to collaborate with those who can see only results. If the determinism implicit in psychology makes it easier to communicate with other professionals, it's nearly impossible to resist.

So there may be fair and good reasons why today's pastoral caregiver may gravitate toward things psychological and away from things spiritual. Even in religious communities, members are much more likely to want help with their issues than with their sin. But, by swallowing some of the historical determinism that is inherent in the psychoanalytic tradition, a caregiver may be trying to speak an objective grammar with a tongue that is incapable of any of the subjective subtleties that make spiritual discourse meaningful.

Inductive Logic Defined

Because so much of our logic is assumed to be deductive, it can be hard to imagine just exactly what inductive logic looks like. In general, it moves in the reverse direction from deductive logic, and by comparison, it has some unexpected qualities.

Part II—Physique and Physics

Mathematics offers a precise definition. A theorem is said to be proved inductively when it is said to be true for any given number, N, and then also true for $N + 1$. The N number is completely random and it represents the completely general. But whereas the N is completely random, the $N +1$ is utterly precise—it is one and only one number different. In other words, when you have an idea that is true in the abstract, and it is also true in the particular, we call that an inductive proof. What gives the inductive proof its movement is the $N + 1$, in many ways analogous to the priming of a pump. Deductive movements usually tend to be based on things we're sure of, as with science. Based on our limited sphere of knowledge we deduce other facts about the subject in question.

We still teach Newton's theory of gravity, even though Einstein was able to predict the force to a greater degree of certainty. But something about the Newtonian world view is more agreeable to us; we like the idea that the universe runs by absolutes, and even though Einstein's relativity is fashionable in today's relative lifestyle, we still prefer to think of things in terms of causes and effects, and that is quintessentially Newtonian. Einstein may currently be in vogue, but Newton is the traditional standard.

It can be hard to imagine the reverse syllogism. Socrates is a man. And there are lots of things that we can say about men—that they have all kinds of limits and boundaries. Maybe we can infer some things about the person of Socrates. But maybe there is something special about Socrates altogether. Maybe he has something new to add to the world. Maybe one human can come along, and not only do something unpredictable—like thinking in a whole new way—but at the same time, change the way all humans think ever after.

Now we are getting close to the essence of the inductive movement. Sometimes, it is the job of the midwife to help the baby come forth. Sometimes the birth process can get stuck and stall. Sometimes the labor must be induced—something must be done either to get things moving, or to change the way things are moving.

Logotherapy

Of course, over the last hundred years, academic psychology has grown and evolved considerably. While it is helpful to consider the historical orientation of psychology towards determinism, there have been many thinkers

Inductive Logic and Being Induced

who developed more dynamic models and a more active appreciation for creativity and the capacity for change.

One branch of psychology that has excelled in the appreciation for human potential has been existential psychology. Psychotherapist Irving Yalom explores some of these very dynamics in his group theory.[1] He articulates the painfully familiar experience of the "vicious cycle" where the experience of failure predisposes the individual toward the likelihood of more failure. A lot of this dynamic is the hallmark of addiction, where failure to resist the addiction results in a loss of self esteem, which creates an even stronger desire to retreat into the addiction. But the pattern is not limited to negative behaviors, and when things get going in the right direction, Yalom uses the concept of the "adaptive spiral" as the *yang* to the *yin* of the "vicious cycle." In short, people who adapt well are even better poised to meet the next challenge successfully. Perhaps this is what is meant by the paradox in Mark when Jesus says "For to him who has will more be given; and from him who has not, even what he has will be taken away" (Mark 4:25).

These paradoxes are part of the human condition, and as scholar Marvin Shaw argues in his book *The Paradox of Intention*, people everywhere have struggled with them. Of greatest interest to the midwife is the current flourishing of paradoxical therapy, of cognitive psychology, and the logotherapy[2] of Victor Frankl. Shaw explains, "Frankl insists this approach is appropriately logotherapy, healing through meaning, because paradoxical intention works without reference to the underlying causes; it is precisely the adopting of a new attitude toward or interpretation of the neurosis."[3]

This begins to approach the Socratic. Socrates did not say that he knew everything: he knew nothing. He did not develop a way of explaining other people's ignorance or a metatheory of how they came to be misinformed. There is a similar thrust in Frankl's work. Here we see a therapy that understands illness dynamically and does not require the idolatry of etiology; that is, where a disease originates is not more important or more emphasized than its cure. Frankl provides a case in point with his own life. He is a concentration camp survivor and he developed logotherapy

---

1. See Yalom and Leszcz, *The Theory and Practice of Group Psychotherapy*, 49.

2. Consider that "psychology" puts the logos at the end of the word and Logotherapy puts it at the front. The therapy is a work that focuses on the intention, ideation, and trajectory of meaning itself. Simply beautiful.

3. Shaw, *The Paradox of Intention*, 71.

Part II—Physique and Physics

as "healing through meaning." The Nazis threatened the meaning of life everywhere, and ultimately, Jewish survival. Frankl chose to interpret this paradoxically: the more death and despair that the Nazis spread, the greater the challenge was to find meaning in life. But that there were such challenges only strengthened his belief in meaning. He writes:

> Life is a task. The religious man differs from the apparently irreligious man only by experiencing his existence not simply as a task, but as a mission. This means that he is also aware of the taskmaster, the source of his mission. For thousands of years that source has been called God.[4]

Ordinarily we usually only see these circular dynamics in the negative. Through paradox Frankl is able to set up a spiritual circular dynamic where the individual is strengthened and edified.

Paradoxical therapy is not some whimsical or poetic response to conflict, but is based on precise principles. Frankl declares, "Paradoxical intention is based on 'the two-fold fact that fear makes come true that which one is afraid of, and that hyperintention makes impossible what one wishes.'"[5] In other words, our fear can develop a spiritual component paradoxically making it seem impossible to avoid the things we want to avoid and being capable of doing the things we want to do.[6] Shaw summarizes this in simpler words, "According to Frankl, we cannot pursue happiness, for if it is our objective, we lose sight of the reason for happiness and happiness itself fades away."[7] As a twentieth-century Jew Frankl understood the greatest threat and paradox to humanity to be meaninglessness. As a response, he developed a method of healing through meaning that has ontological claims about God but ultimately works by means of a paradoxical method.

---

4. Frankl, *The Doctor and the Soul*, xxi.

5. Quoted in Shaw, *The Paradox of Intention*, 71.

6. One is reminded of Paul, writing, "We know that the law is spiritual; but I am carnal, sold under sin. I do not understand my own actions. For I do not do what I want, but I do the very thing I hate. Now if I do what I do not want, I agree that the law is good. So then it is no longer I that do it, but sin which dwells within me. For I know that nothing good dwells within me, that is, in my flesh. I can will what is right, but I cannot do it. For I do not do the good I want, but the evil I do not want is what I do. Now if I do what I do not want, it is no longer I that do it, but sin which dwells within me. So I find it to be a law that when I want to do right, evil lies close at hand. For I delight in the law of God, in my inmost self, but I see in my members another law at war with the law of my mind and making me captive to the law of sin which dwells in my members. Wretched man that I am! Who will deliver me from this body of death?" (Rom 7:14–24).

7. Shaw, *The Paradox of Intention*, 63.

Inductive Logic and Being Induced

Here is a one-liner parable from Frankl: "In general, the leading maxim of existential analysis might be put thus: live as if you were living for the second time and had acted as wrongly the first time as you are about to act now."[8] Frankl positions this maxim to negate both the future mistakes that have not yet happened and the past mistakes that might otherwise constrain us to repeat our mistakes. Instead, the hearer of this parable is invited to participate in life in a new way. Maybe the hearer feels a sense of relief and gratitude that she doesn't have to play out her days by the same old rules and she can choose what she really wants to do. Life becomes less serious, and somehow, the gift of freedom becomes more important and more wonderful.

Frankl uses the term *logotherapy* as a means of treating the meaninglessness of contemporary life. The healing paradox that he throws out is that the more meaningless life becomes, the greater is our duty to find meaning. Our purpose increases by the magnitude of our problem. I would suggest a more broad understanding of logotherapy. In keeping with the Greek root of the word, maybe logotherapy is a therapy of logic. It is a therapy that lets us correct the syntax errors of our lives. By employing the paradox, logotherapy explodes the grammar of the sentences that define who we are. Logotherapy can work in pastoral counseling to explode our personal grammar, just as parables can use paradoxes in literary theory to explode the laws of narrative grammar.

Deductive versus Inductive

Deductive thinking can cultivate a pastoral care that overemphasizes the pathological. Deductive and deterministic approaches focus on the causality of events. What set of conditions and causes led things to be the way they are today? If this person has a problem, where did the problem come from? And this leads to one of the great counterproductive consequences of deterministic pastoral care; instead of being person-centered, it tends to become problem-centered. When things become problem-centered and not person-centered, we stop hearing the stories that people have to tell, and we start looking for some kind of underlying problem. This can really decide the course of what had been a truly open dialogue. When problems and pathologies are the most important thing, that's where we are going to

---

8. Frankl, *The Doctor and the Soul*, 64.

Part II—Physique and Physics

steer a conversation. Understanding the pathology becomes more important than everything, even people. We see what we look for.

On the other hand, inductive logic is much more indeterminate. Instead of assuming the past holds the definitive answer about why things are the way they are, inductive logic is more in tune with how things are moving in the present, and even more so about where things are likely to go in the future. Inductive logic holds out for the possibility of dreaming a new future, and imagining the steps that are necessary to get us there.

In a similar vein, deterministic thought tends to be much more static, whereas inductive thinking is more fluid and dynamic. Deductive thought wants to understand the chain of causality. And that's a noble goal and a reasonable approach, but the approach carries with it a unique set of values. If I think that liberation comes from understanding the past, then I am also placing a high value on conscious comprehension and the ability to understand the past correctly. By valuing conscious comprehension and the ability to understand correctly, we are more and more establishing the ego—that conscious self—as the locus of healing. And that may not be where the healing lies; indeed, the ego can often be the cause of the problem.

By contrast, inductive logic seems better suited to dynamic properties and changing relationships. For instance, two people approaching intimacy are likely to have thoughts and feelings about the intimacy that will affect how they undertake that approach. We are always changing, always in motion, even as that selfsame awareness guides that motion. Instead of trying to find a fixed moment in the past that explains everything, inductive logic is better suited to engage the complexities of the present moment.

Another characteristic of determinism is that the resultant perspective tends to be reductionistic. Determinism looks at broad phenomena and demands to know why. If we all have an experience of love, for example, why does falling in love feel that way? And the deterministic mind sets out for an answer, seeking to understand all of the biological processes that cascade when we fall in love. And finally, we have so dissected the thing that we were originally curious about so that it no longer looks like anything lovely. Mark Twain echoes loudly here: "Humor is like a frog. You can dissect it, but it tends to die in the process."[9] Because determinism wants to understand everything in terms of causal relationships, it tends to reduce wholes into the sum of their parts. Since human beings are physiological

9. Quoted in White and White, eds., *A Subtreasury of American Humor*, xi–xii.

Inductive Logic and Being Induced

organisms, and love is an experience that humans can have, it would also follow that there is a physiological component to the experience of love (hearts race, eyes dilate, etc.). But it does not then follow that falling in love is ultimately a physiological event, much like a rock falling off of a cliff. A hard determinism has an even harder time seeing beyond this, because it is so locked into its vice-like perspective.

Inductive thought can work with abstract truths like love; inductive reasoning is better suited for the objects of faith. It doesn't need to understand love as a biological consequence of evolution. It doesn't need to understand faith as a psychological consequence of evolution (a psychological need of the organism to deny death). Inductive reasoning can accept that faith and love have their own reason for being, and inform how they unfold in the future.

The gravity of formal philosophy settled into deductive logic and determinism, but within mysticism,[10] inductive logic was occasionally embraced and explored. Here's a great example: in introduction to philosophy classes, Anselm is often ridiculed for his "ontological argument of God." The argument suggests that because God is, by definition, the ultimate good, then God must exist because existence itself is a greater good than the idea alone. Determinists laugh and say that Anselm has offered only an immortal example of circular logic. But they miss Anselm's achievement, his purpose, and his context. As an objective argument, meant to convince someone outside the faith, Anselm fails. But as a pious believer, within the context of his faith, the argument succeeds, because it succeeds as an intensifier. Because Anselm has faith that God is good, the argument increases his sense of tangibility of God, because the greatest good would be for God to be tangible. Where the deductive determinist seeks only proof, this inductive mystic seeks movement. The argument is not merely circular, but an upward spiral—and the two-dimensional mind of the determinist cannot measure the vector of inductive reasoning.

---

10. Margaret Guenther offers an interesting tangential reflection. "Even as we are born in the human birth process, so we are born again in our baptism. If Eckhart is to be believed, we give birth and are born ourselves again and again: the birth of God in the soul is our own true birth." With the example of Meister Eckhart, she shows us that mysticism is a place where inductive logic and birthing images have been celebrated. Julian of Norwich would be another place to find feminine images. See *Holy Listening*, loc. 1024–26.

Part III

Immanence and Emanations

PERPENDICULAR TO TRANSCENDENCE, IMMANENCE explores the divinity along horizontal lines. There are obvious resonances with this dialogical medium, dialogue existing between people. Most religions and forms of spirituality have notions of both transcendence and immanence. In Christianity, the word for immanence might be incarnation.

Emanations are helpful because there are many manifestations of the kind of inductive spirituality and indirect movements that we have been describing. I wanted to connect immanence with the concept of emanations because I think they amplify each other.

Chapter 8

Lighting and Dark Sayings

> I will open my mouth in a parable;
> I will utter dark sayings from of old,
> things that we have heard and known,
> that our fathers have told us.
> We will not hide them from their children,
> but tell to the coming generation
> the glorious deeds of the LORD, and his might,
> and the wonders which he has wrought.
>
> PSALM 78:2–4

WE SHOULD NOW HAVE all the tools we need to look at parables in their fullness. So we turn to them as a means of refining theory, and also as a segue of moving the theoretical into the practical. Of course there is an abundance of information and detail that accompanies each parable: historical and sociopolitical context, the rabbinic rhetorical tradition, contemporary philosophic developments, and so on. But the technical form of the parable is so conducive to the gospel that a collective explanation will help us.

The parable comes from the Jewish tradition of the *mashal*, or difficult saying. It is a broader category; it includes proverbs, truisms, aphorisms, and what we usually think of as parables. The Greek phenomena suggests something different. Etymology describes the pairing of two things that are

Part III—Immanence and Emanations

just kind of thrown out there. I like the metaphor of Gary Larson's *Far Side* series, which graced morning newspapers for years with a single image and a single caption. The joke was in the disparity between the two, and often the reader had to work at fitting them together. Remarkably, the parables of a culture otherwise lost to us still hold the weakness and the power to bring us into direct contact with the gospel. But the power of their strangeness has eluded us and on the whole we have set them aside for sermon illustrations and allegories. But the parables have the potential to be powerful inducives for the spiritual midwife. Christianity doesn't need to rely on the school of psychology for all of its tools of pastoral care. Parables can be a good way of returning proclamation to pastoral care—where pastoral care has become afraid of interfering with the individual's self-selected development.

Parables throughout Christianity

Christianity has not always been afraid to parable. One of many shining examples, seventeenth-century thinker Blaise Pascal crafted many parables all for the purpose of Christian upbuilding. He is widely respected for his contributions in several disciplines. Pascal's is an earned reverence; his accomplishments in calculus, his development of an adding machine, and his experiments in physics have secured him a rightful place in the histories of those disciplines. But we turn to his parables.

The most famous is Pascal's Wager. The Wager itself occurs in the *Pensées*, customarily thought to be an apologetic work in progress, never completed. Various editors have compiled, organized, and published the incomplete fragments. This in some sense puts Pascal at a disadvantage, a man who is now eternally caught with his pants down and must square off against every theologian with a penchant for game theory. The "Wager" is actually an untitled pericope beginning with "Infinite—Nothing."[1] It proceeds with a brief exposition on God, infinity, and finitude in the medium most at Pascal's facility: mathematics. It should not be read too seriously as Pascal's final thought on the subject. Numbers are play for Pascal and it is much more likely that Pascal is trying to shrink God down to terms for the rest of us that Pascal is actually straining himself. The Wager then moves into its namesake, a carefully crafted fictional dialectic on "betting" or not betting, an imaginary conversation with a friend stranded in the human

---

1. Pascal, *Selections from the Thoughts*, 86.

Lighting and Dark Sayings

condition: you are going to die. While you're here, are you going to try to establish contact with the one Being who might save you? No? Why not?

Pascal writes, "Let us evaluate these two cases: if you win, you win everything; if you lose, you lose nothing. Wager then without hesitation that he [God] exists."[2] Pascal's emphasis is neither the win/lose dichotomy, nor the existence of God, but the hesitation. There is a way in which we can hold back from walking with God, and there is reason to think that this hesitation is Pascal's tacit aim. Later, in the Wager, he writes about what we can do to help our unbelief. But this is disturbing to us; we sense that the ego is threatened:

> Naturally doing those things will make you believe and will weaken your resistance.
> "But that is what I fear."
> And why? What have you to lose?[3]

His point, as with every parable, is purely polemical and not literal. There is no specific prodigal son and there is no way to fool God with our wagers. But his parable underscores to the speculative reader two things: they have not as yet made such a wager personally; and, assuming all the presupposing formalisms to be true there is no good reason not to wager. Why, then, has the reader not yet wagered? Pascal does not say. He remains respectfully quiet, only saying enough to subtly imply the question.

Wittgenstein is famously quoted as saying, "Whereof one cannot speak, thereof one must keep silent."[4] This book hopes to not say everything that has never been said about that which "one cannot speak." The parables are a map to that inverted world, a map that necessarily looks like an Escher print. Jaspers touches on this when he refers to the communication skills of Socrates and Jesus. He writes, "They express what there is no appropriate way of saying. They speak in parables, dialectical contradictions, conversational replies; they do not fixate."[5] More to the point, he seems to directly address Wittgenstein's proverb: these specific verbal forms of Socrates's irony and Jesus' parables are paradoxically equipped for precisely the phenomena that transcend our language. This is so, as this book hopes to show, because the forms' use of literary negativity destroy the tight links of

2. Ibid., 88.
3. Ibid., 90.
4. Wittgenstein, *Tractatus Logico-philosophicus*, 189.
5. Jaspers, *Socrates, Buddha, Confucius, Jesus*, 90.

comprehension that ordinary positive language relies upon. These negative forms should not be thought of as nonforms that say nothing definitive at all, but these negative forms negate themselves submissively and properly under their mysterious and divine content. Where typical language boldly attempts to name its subject even when the subject is God and there is none greater, these negative forms humbly recognize their limits that we are denied, such as names, and only sketch the faintest lines to show that while it is certain God is (in the fullest sense of the burning bush tradition), there is a boundless expanse to the things we cannot know about God.

The Parables of Jesus

Focusing on parables we encounter a plethora of responses to their intrinsic enigmas. Mark has no qualms about saying that they are deliberately confusing and even off-putting, as Jesus says, "To you has been given the secret of the kingdom of God, but for those outside everything is in parables; so that they may indeed see but not perceive, and may indeed hear but not understand; lest they should turn again, and be forgiven" (Mark 4:11–12). Jaspers comments, "His meaning remains veiled for the unbeliever; to the believer it is revealed, yet even then not in clear statements, but in parables and paradoxes."[6] Even as Jesus is coming clear with all his disciples he manages to do so with tongue in cheek, finding the inclusion of the additional barb irresistible much to the vexation of the twelve, centuries of faithful exegetes, and those of us today who insist that the Christian message is essentially one of being nice and being clearly understood. Where Jesus seems to have welcomed ambiguity and even misinterpretation, we have clearly and eloquently articulated our heresies as we attack the gospel with our language of precision.

For parable scholar John Dominic Crossan, parables work subversively to overturn the established order. In purely literary categories the function of myth is reconciliation. That is, the great archetypal conflicts in life are brought together and reconciled (like developmental myths like Oedipus, where the child must set out on his own against his parents—although there are plenty of reconciliation myths with happier endings than Greek tragedies). Myth reconciles us to the existential facts of life and the needs of contemporary culture (e.g., Camus's brave treatment of the myth of

---

6. Ibid., 71.

Lighting and Dark Sayings

Sisyphus). Crossan is right to say, "Parable brings not peace but the sword, and parable casts fire upon the earth which receives it."[7]

Crossan sees parable at the other end of the dialectical spectrum. The chief function of parable is contradiction.[8] In his words, "Parable is a story which is the polar, or binary, opposite of myth."[9] He describes the relation between myth and parable metaphorically, "You have built a lovely home, myth assures us; but, parable whispers, you are right above an earthquake fault."[10] Crossan's understanding of parable is only similarly negative. His parable is negative only insofar as it plays against type. The ironic parable is intrinsically negative; the negativity is built in. Ironic parable not only subverts the unspoken expectations of the status quo but parable also subverts narrative itself. By turning story inside out, the hearer is able to participate and be drawn in inductively.

Technically, Crossan's parables are marked by the parabolic reversal, which is the moment where the story takes the unexpected turn. This definition is limiting because it requires that the ironic paradox directly weave itself into the narrative fabric. The core parable, for Crossan, becomes the contradiction. Many parables don't lend themselves to this description. Some alleged parables are one-liners, "The kingdom of God is as if a man should scatter seed upon the ground, and should sleep and rise night and day, and the seed should sprout and grow, he knows not how" (Mark 4:26). There is no contradiction for Crossan. Planted seeds tend to grow; nothing subversive there. But what makes it a parable is not the image Jesus uses, but the caption he puts with it; namely, that this ordinary occurrence is like the kingdom of God. Often he is forced to categorically remove the parable out of the parable tradition or to remove it from what is thought to be the genuine body of Jesus' sayings. When parables are considered with regard to irony, the parabolic category widens because the essence of the disparity is not always readily apparent. Sometimes it takes work to find out what or who is being negated. Maybe Jesus' allegories really were allegories and not just parables that the tradition corrupted, because what they negate will depend on who the audience is.

---

7. Crossan, *The Dark Interval*, 38.
8. Ibid., 37.
9. Ibid., 38.
10. Ibid., 40.

89

Part III—Immanence and Emanations

An Ironic Aside

An emerging argument here is that Crossan seems to view the parables two dimensionally, and if the parabolic reversal isn't immediately ready on the page, it must not be a true parable. But what if the parable exists three dimensionally, and engages people that are situated in other ways in the story? Or, what if the parable exists four dimensionally, and works across time itself to the present reader?

The ironic aside comes in because philosophy too has shared this exact debate. Professor Gregory Vlastos[11] in *The Classical Quarterly* has argued that classical irony changed with Socrates and the Platonic dialogues, that before Socrates irony was deceitful (termed simple irony) and that after Socrates irony was wry and humorous (termed complex irony). What is fascinating is the counterpoint that responds to him, and how that counterpoint parallels our critique of Crossan.

Jill Gordon summarizes Vlastos in the following way: "In 'simple' irony what is said is simply not what is meant. In 'complex' irony what is said both is and isn't what is meant."[12] The problem she finds is that there are many other instances of irony, all throughout the dialogues, that are neither accurately captured by Vlastos's definition nor accidental. Paula Gottlieb agrees, especially around the possibility of dramatic irony. She says, "In Plato's hands, Socratic irony takes on an added dimension. For the purposes of dramatic irony, Plato fully exploits the fact that Socratic irony amuses and pleases those in the know, while deceiving and angering those on the outside."[13] With Gottlieb's argument, we begin to recognize a division that we see in the parables; namely, those who have ears to hear and those who do not. These inside and outside divisions created community as they were in inverse proportion to the power structures of the day.

Gordon concludes, "If we ignore the dramatic context of the irony situated in Plato's dialogues we not only unnecessarily exclude too much, but we also ignore an essential aspect of the function of irony. Socratic irony is among the most powerful tools at Socrates's disposal for turning the lives of his interlocutors toward philosophy. And so for Plato and his readers."[14] She makes an important point here: this is not just about Socrates, the Athe-

---

11. Vlastos, "Socratic Irony."
12. Gordon, "Against Vlastos on Complex Irony," 131.
13. Gottlieb, "The Complexity of Socratic Irony," 278.
14. Gordon, "Against Vlastos on Complex Irony," 136–37.

Lighting and Dark Sayings

nians, and his enemies the Sophists. This is about you and me, and anybody else that joins the dialogue.

Hear, Then, the Parable

Parables are a type of existential literature that invite the reader to imaginatively participate. Sometimes they do this by negating the specific and appealing to common experiences. Many people have experiences with sheep or seed in an agricultural society. Sometimes they involve the reader by negating potentiality; they don't cause the hearer to distance themselves from the story by locating it in the hypothetical future (what if a man was going to take a walk on the Sabbath?), but they present themselves in actuality often in the guise of an event that has already begun ("a man went walking from Jerusalem to Jericho") and the final conclusion awaits resolution (as far as we know the brother of the prodigal son is still deciding how to settle his differences). All of this is to say that somehow the main character is negated; the main character is set off into motion before we've been given either a face or name. The only thing of which the hearer is certain is that the story has already started and the main character is "just like me." It would be the same effect of coming in late to a movie about some dimly lit figure coming in late to a movie. Once the hearer is then involved some kind of contradiction begins to unfold. What makes the parable inductive and so applicable in spiritual midwifery is that, like *Monty Python's Holy Grail*, it is only when the lights finally do come up that the viewer realizes the joke is on them.

But back to the parables proper, the first negation is followed by a second negation. We usually find the second negation as a well-crafted literary paradox that has been sewn into the narrative of the parable. Just remember, some of these literary paradoxes are not actually in the parable narrative, but they exist between the audience and the story (as when Jesus is speaking to a group of Pharisees, the paradox may actually be a very transparent story that is spoken to a group with a loaded context).

Therapeutically, inductive theology and parables function quite differently than pop psychology. Where pop psychology seeks to improve our quality of life by helping us resolve seeming conflicts, parable seeks to give us problems. Through parable we are forced to confront the problems of individual life and our social practices. What we see here is a therapy of fiction, parables, and hypothetical cases. So long as the midwife preserves the parables' inherent negativity remembering to stay out of the way, the possibilities for pastoral care are exciting. The midwife is able to conjure just the right character-building predicament and thrust the person into it with a far greater "tailor-made fit" than likely to be encountered in the world at random.

We tend to underestimate Jesus as a logician. We either see Jesus nestled in the context of the Godhead—so supreme and transcendent as to be infinitely above the need of stooping to logic—or we see Jesus as a first-century flat-earther. But within the parables we can easily see a dazzling intelligence and a rhetorical apparatus that is perfectly capable of wielding all the complexity of Socratic irony.

Jesus as Inductive Logician

Ultimately Crossan's emphasis on the parabolic reversal limits the opportunity for ironic interpretation, as only narrative ironies are considered and contextual ironies (location of the speaking event or the particularity of the audience) are ignored. Further, the precise inductive nature of the parable is ignored. Remember the definition of the inductive proof? Crossan's thought represents the N when we all see the truth in a new way, but it fails to appreciate the need for the $N + 1$—that place where this new abstract truth is forced to collide with the particular, the hearer, the individual, you. Parables understood inductively can have several negatives: the main character is negated (so the hearer is induced into the story) and preconceived myths are negated (conventional wisdom explodes in a paradox). This leaves us with an equation to reduce; we are left with the parenthetical elements of the previous sentence. We have the hearer in one hand and the exploding paradox in the other. So now these two things are brought into ironic collision. The hearer is left with this negativity to resolve and work out with fear and trembling. We can understand this induction through irony, mathematics, and theology.

There's something subtle here. Jesus induces the hearer into the parable by means of a first negation (we can think of this move as an N), and then Jesus lets the parable do its life-changing work by means of a second negation (and we can think of this as an $N + 1$). So, in most cases, the first negation is achieved through grammatical mood—that is, the parables are usually cast into the subjunctive. It's no surprise that so many of the characters are unnamed. The hypothetical nature of these parable characters

Lighting and Dark Sayings

increases the sense of the subjunctive—a metaphysical musing, a self-proclaimed fiction, that has very little to do with any of the distracting personage of Jesus. What's really interesting is that many of the parables begin in the past tense, but they end unresolved and pointed into the future (where all of the transformation is going to occur).

Just by way of clarification, Socrates usually works his first negation by tackling his own distracting personage directly. He'll say, "I don't know, and I'm glad to find an expert like you. Please help a foolish old man." Socrates is typically much more self-effacing with the first negation, although there are many times, specifically in Matthew, Mark and Luke, where Jesus practices this kind of personal disavowal. "Don't call me good, only God the Father is good" (Matt 19:17; Mark 10:18; Luke 18:19).

A Significant Footnote

The logic behind that kind of maneuver, the above referenced disavowal of Jesus, deserves some nuance and exposition. There's a lot going on there. Moreover, this technique is modeled repeatedly in John's gospel.

It starts with John the Baptist. The point is almost belabored that John was sent before Jesus because John was not the truth but needed to make way for the truth. What? Why? Why go on and on about someone only for the sake of dismissing them? Why talk so much about John the Baptist only so that we can establish that we are *not* going to talk about John the Baptist?

In programming, there is the concept of the "pointer." The pointer is not a value, but a placeholder that points to an actual value. In mathematics, an important concept is that of substitution, because substitution allows you to replace one complex expression for another. This is abstraction and extrapolation itself, in many ways the essence of all abstract thought. In language, this is a poem—where a series of words and images come to embody a very precise meaning or feeling.

John continues this throughout the Gospel, and Jesus frequently transacts this kind of substitutionary logic. Jesus says things like, "If you have seen me, you have seen the Father" (John 14:19). Here the substitutions point toward God. But Jesus also reverses the flow, rather fluidly, and says things like, "As God has sent me, I send you"—the substitutions here pointing to persons. He uses this logic with his disciples, with his opponents, and it permeates the Gospel. These substitutions echo of Aristotle's syllogisms (if A is greater than B, and B is greater than C, then A is greater than C).

Part III—Immanence and Emanations

These syllogisms are important because of the movement they convey, but remember that Aristotle's flow here has been derived from Socrates. What Aristotle does with argument, Socrates does in conversation with dialogical partners. Socrates modeled the same rhetorical movements between persons, not the abstract values of a syllogism. Next to Socrates's dynamic dialogue, Aristotle seems sluggishly cognitive and theoretically mired. Aristotle thinks; Socrates dances.

Jesus' mastery of this language is powerful. This is especially interesting in John 8:54: "If I glorify myself, my glory is nothing; it is my Father who glorifies me, of whom you say that he is your God." This seems to embody a lot of the maneuvering we have previously described in objective and subjective relationships. If Jesus glorifies himself, that's going to be an ironic collision. That's not going to work and it necessarily must come from another source, perhaps in much the same way that John the Baptist had to bear witness to the Logos and the light.

This is remarkable in the history of ideas and very countercultural. This collides with so much of the theology around graven images, from the Bible to the iconoclasts. In the Old Testament we have emphatic prohibitions against graven images. These scriptures have informed many reform movements. It is a sin to try to symbolize divinity. While it is foolish to presume, presumably this is because human beings are likely to confuse the symbol and the thing that is being symbolized. We all too often idolize our symbols. The weight of this prohibition cannot be overstated. It is implied in the first commandment. And in many ways, it has been understood as a caution against this kind of abstraction, integrative thought, and symbolic thinking especially around God. We have to keep the Spirit from being confused with the physical things that we use to represent that Spirit.

Philosophers and theologians have had much to say on the problem of graven images. Martin Buber rightly stresses the significance of the fact that God is not an object to be talking about, but the Ultimate Subject Whom we may address. Buber is a Jewish theologian who is trying to preserve the subjective relationship (to borrow Kierkegaard's language) between theologians and their God. Jean Baudrillard in his groundbreaking work *Simulations and Simulcra* explores what happens when we get lost in our graven images—we lose touch with reality and become ensnared in a world of illusion, fantasy, and facsimile.

Lighting and Dark Sayings

Buber and Baudrillard are not lightweights. In each of their contexts, they are exactly right. Beyond these philosophers, the historical moral and cultural force of this tradition against graven images has been massive.

All of this is challenged by the mere rhetorical logic Jesus uses. He seems to feel no constraint in the kind of logic he wields. These fears of symbolizing the divine find no place. And with this radical logic, Jesus seems to suggest that even the value of avoiding false idols, that very value itself, can become its own false idol.

Let's look at how he does it. Sometimes, Jesus is able to engraft a single image with the entire logic of a full parable. Later, also in John, Jesus says,

> When a woman is in travail she has sorrow, because her hour has come; but when she is delivered of the child, she no longer remembers the anguish, for joy that a child is born into the world. So you have sorrow now, but I will see you again and your hearts will rejoice, and no one will take your joy from you (John 16:21–22).

He sets up the logic so that the travail of childbirth becomes a pointer to a deeper joy. He creates this substitution, but it doesn't end there. He maps it to the current experience of the disciples. Except that the map is not one-to-one, it's not a direct reference. It's not like the Greek allegories that so clearly describe the world as we know it. No, it's an inverted and a parabolic reference. He maps his presence with the disciples (which is presumably joyful) to the time of pain and confusion for the mother. He then takes her time of joy and maps it to the unknown future—the *aporia*, the mysterious. More accurately, for the disciples this is unknown and mysterious; for the Christian audience this is not mysterious at all—this is the dark and uncertain space of Holy Saturday. So, Jesus uses the movement of substitution to create an empty space in the expectation of the disciples. Because that space must remain empty it becomes an untouchable hope. And for this great, untouchable hope of all hopes—the resurrection itself—Jesus attaches the eternal tenor to the vehicle of the birthing mother.

Chapter 9

The Center

> The space between heaven and earth is like a bellows.
> The shape changes but not the form;
> The more it moves, the more it yields.
> More words count less.
> Hold fast to the center.
>
> LAO TZU

THERE IS A SPIRITUAL core to midwifery. Margaret Guenther writes, "The Psalmist declares: 'Yet it was you who took me from the womb; you kept me safe on my mother's breast. On you I was cast from my birth, and since my mother bore me you have been my God' (Ps. 22:9–10). We are reminded that the midwife helps new life into being and protects it; even more than the mother, she is the tender guardian of its safety."[1] But how are we to arrive at that spiritual core?

There is one more powerful idea that is helpful in learning about spiritual midwifery, and that is the notion of "the center." The center is ultimately a subjective concept, and one that would be impossible to completely define objectively. It is an idea that does not rest in other ideas. It is a term that brings other terms into definition and therefore is impossible to define with those selfsame other words. To describe it, we must test the tensile strength of our language and reach with a sense of the poetic.

---

1. Guenther, *Holy Listening*, loc. 1003–7.

The Center

At the same time, just because the center cannot be defined by precise terms does not mean that we cannot talk about it, that we cannot talk around it, that we cannot circumambulate the truth like a labyrinth, that we cannot be made better by it even as we struggle to understand it. A term does not have to be completely pinned down in order to be useful. By now, we know we can find many needful things that are necessarily subjective, if we are willing to walk subjectively.

Embedded in this conversation is a twin notion of paradox. We have been exploring the kind of energy and movement that exists between persons, especially in dialogue. We have been alluding to the great common ground that exists between people, and which is the mutual half-step of compromise and the beginning of change. Theologians may have the market on the "now and not yet" but it is midwifery that governs the territory between them. There is also a sense in which this great conceptual center also mirrors and relates to the very centering of the heart of the midwife.

Moving toward the center requires that the conversation move toward the heart of dialectical theory and a greater appreciation of formal dialectics. We have explored relationships and the dialectical tension that often characterizes them. Dialectics lie at the core of midwifery, and the movement of the individual at the paradox of the parable moves by dialectical principles. When a person meets the double negativity of Socrates or Jesus, how can we understand the resulting movement to follow? Through dialectics. Remember that Socrates's rare metaphor was the "spiritual midwife." His ordinary term of choice seems to have been *dialectician*.

Dialectics have played a powerful role in philosophy and religion from the very beginning, and Heraclitus did a lot of the initial pioneering of dialectics in the West. Heraclitus spoke about the great juxtaposition of life, the war between here and there, now and then, dualism against dualism, and as the mystic Heraclitus suggests, the very universe is suspended in a great dialectical tension. Most of human spirituality has had a great respect for the primary dualisms, antinomies, and binary opposites that mark life as we know it—and it is through a dialectical process that spirituality is able to transcend them. By exploring dialectics we begin to understand the empty spaces and negative spaces that are described by Lao Tzu. We begin to think about using the space that is not there.

And while this is the trajectory we are headed for, the great in-between of everything, the center of the center, we can also surrender to the fact that we don't have to comprehend the greatest mysteries in order to appreciate them. There are some very abstract and lofty dimensions to dialectical thought, but while the dialectical principle can turn the mind outward, it can also turn the mind inward. This very abstract and remote thought can have a personal feel. We begin to understand the universal dialectic and the great dialectic between persons, through all of its forms and manifestations of dialogue, but now we turn to the inner experience of dialectic within a person—and in this case that is the person of the midwife.

It is profoundly obvious why a midwife would need to be centered. Mother is going through a crisis that will change her life. She is going through the cataclysm of being. It is a process that will result in a life or a death, a dynamic process that is not guaranteed. Not only is it the birth of a child, but it is the becoming of a parent. It is the beginning of a family. It is a familiar pattern begun from the beginning of time, but it is about to begin for the first time. And in faithfully remaining in this pattern of regular birth, life achieves its dynamic vitality and revitalization.

The last thing a midwife needs to be is scattered. Much of what she needs to do is instill a sense of peace and purpose in the room. There is a lot of energy in the room, energy that is there for a purpose. That energy is going to have to be harnessed and focused and not diffuse if it is going to do its job.

Not only is it important to the mother that the midwife is centered, it is also paramount and directive to the midwife. A sense of the center not only soothes everyone in the room, but it helps the midwife know what to do and when to do it. It is in being still, watchful, and ready that the midwife is able to make the right intervention at the right time. It is this center that guides the midwife and informs her movements. The center becomes a dynamic guide, able to say both "a little to the left" and "a little to the right" at the same time. Because the center is categorically in the dialectical midst of everything, poised at the dialectical heart, it is sensitive and responsive to the slightest imbalance and simultaneously eternally patient enough to let things take their course.

What the Center Is Not

The center is not an external idea or group of ideas like a doctrine that can be superimposed over a relationship in order to bring structure or lessen anxiety. Being centered cannot happen by sheer force of will.

The Center

The center is not an experience where all of the concerns of the midwife disappear—as though the midwife were no longer a person who had concerns and cares. It is more that the center is a place where the midwife can exist as a whole person without threat or anxiety.

The center is not something to be chased after like a balancing act. We have described a lot of different traits or characteristics that need to remain in dialectical tension. When these tensions sometimes collapse, it can feel like a lot of rebalancing, shifting, and juggling are necessary. Maybe so, but this is not the center. It is nearly impossible to find the center whenever it becomes an externalized target outside the self. If you're thinking about hitting a target, you are creating distance away from the center. Centering comes first. Balancing comes second.

Being centered is not a cognitive or rational project. Having some kind of theory of being centered is nice, but it won't achieve that for you. There are differences between understanding water and hydration, being thirsty, and being satisfied. Of the three experiences, being centered might be the closest to fasting.

Being centered is not being scattered. It is not needing the approval of the people that you are trying to midwife. It is not needing to reveal everything you know. It is certainly not needing to be understood. It is not needing to have something to say. It is not needing to appear smart. It is not needing to appear anything. It is not even needing to appear.

What the Center Is

Being centered is being free to be oneself without tripping over oneself. This is very much the way musicians and dancers are able to do the rather ordinary miracles that they do. If they really stopped and thought about all of the individual movements, these achievements could never happen. But they are certainly aware of what they are doing.

The center is the vantage point from which to watch people suffer.

It is also the vantage point from which to watch the sun rise and transformation unfold.

Being centered is a kind of readiness for the business of midwifery. No one's going to hand you their baby if they think you are going to drop it. Nor should they. Being centered is an implicit willingness to hold something, to receive something, not because that's the order of things, but because that's part of the dynamic trajectory of the process.

It is comfortable with being helpless and useless; it is also ready to act. Being centered is both spontaneous and impatient, impulsive and restrained, ready to pull the trigger and not trigger-happy. Take the big leap or walk away.

Like many things, it goes without saying.

It is purposeful without an agenda. It has goals that emanate from the other.

There is a sense of being engaged and involved in what's going on, but also a sense of detachment; being real, but also being real clear about where the focus belongs. Because the midwife is a whole person, there is no need to work on personal problems at the wrong time. Personal problems get their attention, and so there is no distraction. This doesn't come through compartmentalization, but integration.

Being centered is an ideal place to be working with these dialectical in-betweens. It takes a keen focus and a strong determination to resist the polar extremes. Dualism is really built into the human condition and we often live in bifurcations and false dichotomies. There's a lot of safety at the polar extremes because there are a lot of people already there, so it has to be a choice to see other alternatives and find another way.

It might be the peace that passes all understanding, because understanding is largely overrated.

The center is something to trust in. Trust is contagious, inductively.

Becoming Centered

Becoming centered is a process. It doesn't happen all at once. Failures are a part of the process, although dynamically speaking, failures can both take you away from being centered or take you closer to it. The good news is that being centered is much, much easier than being enlightened, and most people can have an experience of being centered if they really want it and are willing to work at it for some time.

Most people find the center by realizing they are not there. That's part of it. You learn to make peace with the distances between you and the center, and the more the anxiety about not being centered lessens, the smaller the distances become. If you want to find the center, you are going to have to spend some significant time not being centered. That's got to be okay.

The Center

Being centered ebbs and flows. There are good days and bad. The person who experiences being centered is still very much human and is still subject to the same forces that buffet us all.

Becoming centered is the central interior practice. It is worth remembering to do, and certainly much more worthy than a lot of the anxious, self-destructive self-talk that is too easy to make time for.

Being centered is not prayer, but has some analogous qualities to prayer. It doesn't make prayer "better" because "better" doesn't really apply to prayer, but it is an interesting space to pray from.

Confidence is the first step toward bringing the catalyst of faith into the room.

Chapter 10

Precepts, Forceps, and Applications

> But nobler far is the serious pursuit of the dialectician,
> who, finding a congenial soul,
> by the help of science sows and plants therein words
> which are able to help themselves and him who planted them,
> and are not unfruitful,
> but have in them a seed
> which others brought up in different soils render immortal,
> making the possessors of it
> happy to the utmost extent of human happiness.
>
> Plato,
>
> PHAEDRUS

> Jesus said: Look, the sower went out,
> he filled his hand (and) cast (the seed).
> Some fell upon the road; the birds came, they gathered them.
> Others fell upon the rock, and struck no root in the ground,
> nor did they produce any ears. And others fell on the thorns;
> they choked the seed and the worm ate them.
> And others fell on the good earth, and it produced good fruit;
> it yielded sixty per measure
> and a hundred and twenty per measure.
>
> Gospel of Thomas,
>
> BLATZ TRANSLATION

Precepts, Forceps, and Applications

IN MY INITIAL RESEARCH, I came across the work of the famous horse trainer, Monty Roberts, and his memoir *The Man Who Listens to Horses*. Roberts is the first "horse whisperer" to publish his method to the world. Roberts does not focus on people at all but primarily works with horses. I struggled with the inclusion of this material for various reasons. But I later discovered something astounding. Socrates had three main biographers and most of our understanding comes from Plato, but another disciple was Xenophon, and Xenophon is said to be antiquity's first horse whisperer. His treatise on horses does not describe anything like the Socratic midwifery—although he does describe the need to be very attentive to the horse and attuned to equine behavior. Still, the dynamics of Roberts's method are profoundly, classically, dialectical.

Roberts's accomplishment is remarkable. So in much the same way as scientists use animal research to help our understandings of humanity, I would like to make brief mention of Roberts's work. Additionally, he has gone the extra distance and used these techniques in working with people, both troubled youth or other trainers. He also remarks that people who have been abused or coerced often have profound reactions to his techniques; it is not uncommon for bystander abuse victims to faint at his horse demonstrations—people who are doing nothing more than observing.

Roberts is actually able to create an intentional and purposeful relationship between a person and an animal. Horses are herd animals and very social. He explains, "The horse is the quintessential flight animal. When pressure is applied to the relationship, he will almost always choose to leave rather than fight."[1] Perhaps their extreme sociability paired with an extreme desire to avoid conflict makes them more like humans than might first seem the case. At any rate, Roberts has had the opportunity to study their social cues and methods of communication. While horses were formerly "broken" into submission through fear and often bloody violence, Roberts creates a trusting relationship through a method of "starting" the horse. In a peaceful meeting of only half an hour to an hour, Roberts is miraculously able to achieve results that are more effective than weeks of traditional horsebreaking. The time differential is no exaggeration—in an hour Roberts can saddle and ride a horse for the first time. His secret? He writes, "The first rule of starting a fresh horse, then, is *no pain*."[2]

---

1. Roberts, *The Man Who Listens to Horses*, 278.
2. Ibid., 278.

Part III—Immanence and Emanations

There are several things that Roberts is accomplishing. His entire theory is not built on etiology or the pathology of spiritual illness, but built on love and respect. It makes sense that this foundational block is "no pain." Another accomplishment is that by refusing to resort to violence he preserves a basic equality in the relationship. Many counseling relationships, either in psychology or pastoral care, have a downward direction where the help flows from the expert to the ignorant.

Further, what he says specifically about pain is crucial. Of course it is obvious not to punish or condemn the counselee, but often times psychotherapy sets out to superimpose itself over the person's previous psychic injuries either positively (e.g., learning how to reframe things through cognitive therapy) or negatively (e.g., learning how to cast off inappropriate guilt and shame that may have come through abuse). But in either case the therapy hopes to supersede the problems. That is worth highlighting: there are theological objections to a type of pastoral care where the goal is for the therapy (or therapist) to supersede the "problem." Besides, it is incredibly difficult to transplant one set of experiences for another. Kierkegaard knew this when he described his theory of literary communication: "No, an illusion can never be destroyed directly, and only by indirect means can it be radically removed."[3] And Roberts knows that pain in horsebreaking has one purpose: to make the horse forget everything it has known about social interaction and to recognize the trainer as the supreme authority. My emphasis is meant to suggest that trying to replace one set of experiences and reflexes over atop another may not only be needlessly inefficient but also somehow violent. In the therapeutic setting this is evident when counselors encourage counselees to shout, cry, or whatever when the counselor tells the patient how to express their feelings.

More specifically, Roberts's technique works through what he calls Advance and Retreat. He adds, "The phenomenon that I call Advance and Retreat is evident throughout the animal kingdom—between animals of the same and different species and even between humans."[4] Simply, it is a method of expressing social interest in a horse and then withdrawing that interest to communicate likes and dislikes about the horse's behavior. The method is different from other types of reward/punishment systems because there the aim is the manipulation of a set of behaviors. Here, the aim always has the relationship to the animal fresh in mind. And the dis-

---

3. Kierkegaard, *The Point Of View*, 24.
4. Roberts, *The Man Who Listens to Horses*, 278.

Precepts, Forceps, and Applications

tinction pays: the horse comes to want to please you more than to eat the carrot on the end of the stick. Advance and Retreat might be the most elementary type of spiritual midwifery; the technical principle would be that the trainer is creating a type of relational negativity, where the other now feels at liberty to enter and come forth. It certainly echoes of the ministry of absence.

The final component of Roberts's method that I would like to isolate is his steady admonition to watch carefully and stay calm. He advises, "Do not rush matters."[5] The spiritual midwife enters into one of the most sensitive relationships with the person who labors. They will invariably perceive any kind of impatience or anxiety, and this in turn will compound the birthing process. In Roberts's scenario you run the risk of spooking the horse and if you are clumsy enough you can scar the animal.

Roberts has provided an example of applied relational negativity for the purpose of creating a therapeutic relationship. He has done so at the scale that serves as clinical research and provides a venue where the ideas herein are manifested and not just ethereal and abstract. Quite independently of academic philosophy, Roberts has developed a sophisticated and articulate method of relating to others that necessarily transcends verbal communication. And most importantly, he has done so successfully.

Still, for those of us who don't frequent stables, but find ourselves out in the wild, here are some suggestions for the application of spiritual midwifery.

Prayer

The midwife is encouraged to pray for the individual in preparation to meet. Pray for them in their absence that you might be absent in their presence. Pray that you will not find service a thing to be grasped, but that you will empty yourself, taking on the form of a servant, becoming obedient in all things—even obedient unto silence. When you are with them, try not to pray on their behalf—distinguishing between prayers that are for them and prayers that might accidentally supersede theirs. Don't be afraid of silences; you can even pray silently with them there. We think of prayer as a very intimate hiding away with God. By definition, three persons tend to be too much of a crowd for dialogical intimacy. The hope is for the midwife to become transparent in the prayer, translucent and nearly invisible, leaving

---

5. Ibid., 284.

Part III—Immanence and Emanations

only God and the individual together in privacy. Think outside the box; it is not inappropriate to say, "I'm going to leave you and God alone for a few minutes," and then leave. They're going to be living the rest of their lives alone with God, and the sooner they get used to the idea the better. If they consistently want you to lead the prayer, consider negating yourself by asking them to pray for you. Encourage them to find the words.

But at times your neighbor will have no words. At those times we count on the greater community to be faithful for us. Prayer books and creeds are a priceless resource here. The midwife can pray and lead the prayer in an outward sense, but inwardly the midwife doesn't lead the prayer at all. The words are starkly there on the page and we read them and pray them because the tradition hands them down to us. The Psalms and the rest of the Bible can be used in this way through the tradition of the *lectio divina*, sometimes very particularly with specific reference to named struggles—but the midwife remains hidden—hidden behind the dash, and behind God's Word.

More personally, there are many instances where the spiritual midwife may want to lead a prayer. One feature of Christian prayer in particular is that it is paradox-making. Some classical paradoxes are that God is all powerful and all loving, that Jesus is fully God and fully human, that Jesus was a man who died and is returned from the grave. The very act of prayer brings us into contact with paradoxes. Even though we continue to sin, we hold to the faith that prayer can change us. Even though day after day we continue to face "unanswered prayer," we hold to the faith that prayer changes God. The Apostles' Creed stands as a good collection of paradoxes. And most of the heresies were formed when people could no longer abide the tension of the contradiction. Because the inconceivability of the God-man was too much to bear, the Docetists found it much more tolerable to say that God was not fully human. We do the same thing in our prayers, although more often through the things we are afraid to pray for. It is as if we cannot bear the pain of holding the doctrine and the disappointment.

Prayer is intimate and vulnerable but also creative. When we pray we are participating in God's creative act—not in the sense that through prayer we are able to influence God in the outcome of creation, but that we are experiencing the gift of naming things just as Adam experienced the gift in Genesis. Although two-way communication in prayer is by no means impossible, insofar as God has granted us the privilege to speak, God has also promised to keep silent. Prayer is partially our chance to use our words and consecrate our thought within the silent space that God provides. In that silence we may express the paradoxical nature of the tumultuous human condition.

Prayer is the place where, in faith, the paradoxes of the faith are set forth. Paradoxes are good ways of expressing things that we really don't have words for. Prayer is faithful when it sets out the paradoxes that anxiety would have us resolve. We do this whenever we encounter mysteries of the faith and rewrite them so they are explicable to us, as with biblical miracles. But praying faithfully means that we pray for the miracle, especially when it doesn't look good, not because we have learned that prayer is a technology for controlling nature, but because we have learned that prayer is a place for speaking the truth, even when the truth sounds funny and alien to our ears. The purpose in making paradoxes in prayer is not to convince ourselves of things we don't believe (although there certainly is merit in that for the embryonic faith) or to insist that God will ultimately conform to human wishes and that God's will shall be revealed in accordance with our own. But these paradoxes create space for God, just as the tools of irony create space for the birthing spirit. Through this kind of prayer the individual learns how to begin relating to God.

Questions

Questions are a significant issue for spiritual midwifery. B. Preston Bogia is right to say, "Questions present a tricky and sometimes awkward situation for a counselor."[6] After all at first it might seem like questions are crucial to the midwife's project. As Diogenes Allen points out, "The midwife puts nothing into a mother but helps her deliver what is within her. By his questions Socrates stimulates another person to discover what is within and finally to deliver the right answer."[7] Kierkegaard summarizes that Socrates uses questions in a qualified way:

> That is, one can ask with the intention of receiving an answer containing the desired fullness, and hence the more one asks, the deeper and more significant becomes the answer; or one can ask without any interest in the answer except to suck out the apparent

6. Bogia, "Responding to Questions in Pastoral Care," 357.
7. Allen, *Philosophy for Understanding Theology*, 41.

Part III—Immanence and Emanations

content by means of the question and leave an emptiness behind. The first method presupposes, of course, that there is a plenitude; the second that there is an emptiness. The first is a *speculative* method; the second the *ironic*. Socrates in particular practiced the latter method.[8]

Bogia continues, "Generally speaking, questions possess two characteristics: they demand answers, and they put one on the defensive."[9] The context of the question is the circumstances under which the person has come to the midwife and the balance of power between them. In Kierkegaard's words, "To ask questions denotes in part the individual's relation to the subject, in part the individual's relation to another individual."[10] Usually, before the first question is ever asked, the person is already in a vulnerable and powerless place. The counselee has no power.[11]

For this reason, because of what it means to assume the helping role, Bogia writes, "*Questions asked by the counselor are almost always experienced as an attack, intrusion, demand.*"[12] While Bogia's comment has the counselor in mind, we must recalibrate it for the greater responsibility of the pastoral role. Whatever authority the counselor has, the pastor has infinitely more. The pastor is more subject to all kinds of projections and transferences. Every previous clerical, parental, and even gender-based relationship can be confused with what is offered in the helping role. Therefore the pastor has a great need to self-negate through irony. To correct the awkwardness in the counselor's questions, Bogia makes several suggestions. Bogia's concern is to avoid questions and in their place use statements of observation and personal preference. Nonverbal communication can be helpful. Even imperatives can be more helpful than the deafening negativity of questions. Bogia writes, "A statement like, 'Tell me more about your father' leaves the counselee free to choose the information that seems important to reveal. The general area of interest has been defined, but what is said is left to the person who is seeking help."[13]

---

8. Kierkegaard, *The Concept of Irony*, 36.
9. Bogia, "Responding to Questions in Pastoral Care," 357.
10. Kierkegaard, *The Concept of Irony*, 34.
11. Bogia, "Responding to Questions in Pastoral Care," 358.
12. Ibid., 359.
13. Ibid., 361.

Precepts, Forceps, and Applications

Bogia also suggests that *"Questions asked by the counselee are almost always intended to convey a message."*[14] Here he makes the suggestion that we should strive to respond to the question instead of answering it. The spiritual midwife is wary of quick and easy answers. The tension behind such questions is intrinsic to the birthing process; the patient's questions are part of the birth pangs. As mentioned, questions are composed to be vague—they deliberately position many rare and specific words around the terrible vagary of an unknown chasm. When we answer a question like this, as if the patient asks, "What if I die?," the result of a direct answer is like shooting an arrow into the Grand Canyon. The trouble is that the answer is likely to miss the mark. The midwife is encouraged to really listen to the question, and then draw the individual out into that chasm, so she can begin to define its limits for herself. It took that person a lifetime to ask that question; try not to answer it in ten words or less.

Prorsus Credibile Est, Quia Ineptum Est
It's to Be Believed Because It's Absurd

It doesn't take much. With just a few words stitched into a secret, Tertullian launches the inconceivable. The paradox before us is palpably sharp and pointed. The Absurd. Who can believe such a thing?

Tertullian himself became absurd when he whispered those words into eternity's ear. With little more than a flick of his wrist and the Spirit that swelled in his heart, he cut the words once and for all into the paper and into the soul of the church. In that brief moment, that slippery instant where thoughts melt away and only letters are left standing, the subject and predicate fused into one and he became a fool for the gospel. In becoming a fool for the gospel, he became a fool for eternity. This does not sit well with us. It is far too reckless; it strikes us as devoid of the calculus to which we cling for survival every day. We calculate each day as we navigate through life, thus reducing things to the simplest factors of what we really need, what we really want, and the most reasonable way to get more out of life for less.

Rather than revere him, we might rather like to rescue Tertullian, we might like to find some way to reach back and excuse his ignorance. We are embarrassed by him and embarrassed for him. We see him as

14. Ibid., 368.

Part III—Immanence and Emanations

being impaled on his ignorance, nailed to this cross by pre-Enlightenment stupidity. We might like to offer him an excuse or two, a chance to benefit from the last 1,800 years of advancement in human thought. Perhaps if he had the benefit of our wisdom he might have said otherwise. We might like to advise him of our psychology and science, or maybe our medicine or our literary criticism. But as yet, Tertullian has not been tempted away from his absurd. Instead he stands firm forever; forever denying our disgrace of excuses. No, he made his choice once and for all and stands with it. He chose the Absurd and meant to do so. There is an inductive movement imbedded within Tertullian's words. The absurdity precedes the belief, and then in turn it is the belief that transcends the absurd. But it is almost as if the absurd beckons the belief.

In Tertullian's case, this turns out to be something very Christian: the Trinity itself—which term Tertullian coined—is an impressive piece of dialectical theology. But there is something even deeper here: perhaps the heart of all spirituality and the very nature of faith. Faith itself reaches out into that space that cannot be touched.

This work could have been called anything. We could have called it "Resistance Based Therapy" (for much of spiritual midwifery is about the overcoming of resistance) and given it an acronym like RBT. Position it next to a few coiffured statistics and numbers, and we could have called it a study, and it probably would have cast a much larger shadow.

But that's not the point.

The point is that these older streams of philosophy and religion have something to stand behind. They stem from a much older and broader source.

But let's forget this confusing muddle and turn back to Tertullian, who so successfully achieved what today we would consider an embarrassment. It seems Tertullian is absurd because he believes in the Absurd. And that is something we are less and less able to do these days. It seems now that we are only able to believe in something that we understand. It is as though we have lost all language that might enable us to talk about the unspeakable. What we believe has become synonymous and limited to our comprehension. We believe the sum of two and two to be four because we understand it and grasp it, and we reach out to the mysteries and absurdities of life with the same small, tight hand. To do as Tertullian has done is now unthinkable. Being "thinkable" is the prerequisite to "believable." Believable in the old sense is something we are able and willing to live out, something we

Precepts, Forceps, and Applications

are willing to shape our lives around. In more common parlance belief is something to which we give intellectual assent. In either sense, rationality has become key to our belief. We are not willing to identify ourselves with or in any way endorse anything irrational, and we certainly wouldn't dedicate our lives (the original meaning of belief) to anything so unreasonable as the Absurd.

But what is most important is not that Tertullian believes in the Absurd, because his quote doesn't say that at all, but that he believes because it is absurd. Tertullian believes in the Absurd, yes, and in so doing achieves something that is lost to us today. But this achievement is on Tertullian's part almost an accident. It is a side effect at best and probably one that passed his age unnoticed. No one would have seen someone who believed in the absurd in the midst of a prefactual world. Fact was a currency that was not yet minted.

Absurdity, here, is alluring. Absurdity is intriguing. Enticing. Inductive. It points to something and takes us there.

Beyond any shame and the threat of being foolish, Tertullian bravely stands without any control at all. But it goes against everything we trust to believe in the Absurd.

He believes because it is absurd. It is this single idea that might be the most powerful inducive of all. Jesus says, "You believe because you have seen; blessed are those who believe and have not seen" (John 20:29). Paul says, "We look not to the things that are seen, but to the things that are unseen" (2 Cor 4:18). Kierkegaard says, "What I am seeking is not here, and for that very reason I believe it."[15] Heraclitus says, "He who cannot seek the unforeseen is lost, for the known way is an impasse."[16]

The real strength of Tertullian's move is that he believes because it is absurd. It is precisely because he can't wrap his mind around the divine paradox that he just might be onto something. When a twentieth-century Jewish architect was commissioned to construct a Christian church in Ohio, he designed it in such a way so that all of the angles and points of convergence met in space; they met well beyond the scope of the church. Rather than gothic cathedrals that try to actually encapsulate God by making God's house sufficiently large, this little church would prefer to be sufficiently small. In so doing it points at, but never goes so far as to name, the largeness of God. The contrast in architecture reveals that, while lacking

---

15. Kierkegaard, *Upbuilding Discourses in Various Spirits*, 218.
16. Heraclitus, *Fragments*, 7.

Part III—Immanence and Emanations

grandiosity, the use of understatement, unresolved paradoxes, and hanging tensions can say things and express truths more honestly and clearly. Because it is absurd.

Afterward and Afterword

The Symposium

O N JUNE 22, 2012 at Capital Health, the hospital where I serve in Trenton, New Jersey, we hosted an event called "The Symposium for Spiritual Midwifery." The Symposium was an all-day event, funded through a grant as a Pastoral Study Project of the Louisville Institute. The support of the Institute has been invaluable, especially the thoughtful comments of Don Richter.

We gathered together a group of scholars from surrounding seminaries and institutions of the New Jersey area. In manuscript form, we discussed the book you are now reading at length, its various flaws and strengths, and some of the ideas behind the book. I'll let the speakers introduce themselves:

Tim Pretz: "I am an ordained minister in the Presbyterian Church, PCUSA. I have served for twenty-one years in two pastorates with a growing interest in working with marriages, so I received some more training and eventually became a clinical member of AAMFT (American Association of Marriage and Family Therapy), and transitioned from pastoral ministry to counseling about eleven years ago. I am an affiliate instructor at Palmer Seminary, which is connected with Eastern University. So I work in pastoral ministries and pastoral counseling in addition to my private practice in marriage and family therapy."

Storm Swain: "I teach at the Lutheran Theological Seminary of Philadelphia. I was ordained as an Anglican priest in New Zealand and am now an Episcopal priest over here and have a background in general hospital and primarily psychiatric chaplaincy. I came and did my doctorate at Union Theological Seminary and my clinical training at Blanton Peale Institute."

Debbie Davis: "I graduated from Princeton Theological Seminary. I was a chaplain—hospital chaplain and nursing home chaplain—for twenty-eight years, Director of the Department at Princeton Hospital, and for the last five years I have been the Director of Field Education at Princeton Theological Seminary."

Johann Vento: "I teach at Georgian Court University in Lakewood, New Jersey. It's a small Catholic women's college run by the Sisters of Mercy, and we just announced we're going coed. We also have a graduate program in theology that focuses on pastoral ministry, primarily parish ministry. My background is in systematic theology."

Will Ashley: "Currently, and for the next thirty days, I'm Director of Field Education and tenured associate professor of Practical Theology at New Brunswick Seminary. In thirty days I'll become the academic dean at the seminary. I'm currently the president of the central New Jersey chapter of the AAMFT. I'm a Blanton Peale graduate, and I've been a pastor for thirty years."

Barbara Chaapel: "I'm, I think like you, Johann, the other one here who has no background in this—hospital or clinical pastoral education (CPE). I'm a minister in the Presbyterian Church USA, have been a college chaplain at Dickinson College, and was Debbie Davis's chaplain at Dickinson. Then, I was called to be a pastor at a large congregation outside of Philadelphia in Bryn Mawr. I still live in Philadelphia. Currently, I'm the Communications Director at Princeton Seminary. I've been there for thirty-one years, I think, and I'm also a parish associate minister at First Presbyterian Church in Philadelphia."

Arthur Pressley: "I teach pastoral care at Drew Seminary. I'm a clinical psychologist. I do a lot of testing and work with children and clergy. I do a lot of work with trauma. I have pastored churches in the Apostolic tradition, and I've pastored Methodist churches, but that was a few years ago."

It is also important to mention a few others who were there. They were my CPE trainees: George Akins III, Sylvester Ekunwe, Ebb Hagan, Bora Kim, Charles Milton, John Schneider, and Aaron Twitchell. I'm thankful to all of these for their spirit, support, and help, especially Aaron who undertook many of the details of the day. I also want to thank Matthew Rhodes for helping to sort through the notes of the Symposium and Amber Carlson with further research. My wife, Heather, was there, and she brought our

The Symposium

children, too. Dan Casselberry, from Pennington United Methodist where I am appointed, was also there.

It was a beautiful day. A typical bright, humid day in June. At the end of the day we shared a meal. The meal was followed by a true symposium, and we tried to pattern the event after Plato's *Symposium*. Plato's *Symposium* is a philosophical drinking party, where all the guests shared a speech on Love. I had invited each guest to prepare their own speech on the book. The subject was wide open. It could be a tangential thought or a direct contradiction. Whatever they wanted to engage me on. I felt like they had been subjected to my thoughts, and they could respond in whatever creative way they wanted.

We quickly established our own drinking rules, and charted our course for the evening. I always feel funny to offer grace over a meal in a room full of clergy. So, I offered two reflections. Each reflection was a synthesis of the words of Diotima and Paul. Diotima is an interesting character. There were no women at Plato's *Symposium*. But Socrates invokes her wisdom. He says that she's the one who taught him the art of love. It strikes me as a perfect negation, to defer to the wisdom of the one woman not there.

In describing eternal beauty, she offers the following:

> First, . . . it always *is*
> and neither comes to be nor passes away,
> neither waxes nor wanes.
> Second, it is not beautiful this way and ugly that way,
> nor beautiful at one time and ugly at another,
> . . . it is itself by itself with itself, it is always one in form;
> and all the other beautiful things share in it,
> in such a way that when those others come to be or pass away,
> this does not suffer any change . . . .
> The love of the gods belongs to anyone
> who has given birth to true virtue and nourished it,
> and if any human being could become immortal,
> it would be he.[1]

I felt a very similar sentiment in Paul:

> Love is patient, love is kind.
> It does not envy, it does not boast, it is not proud.

---

1. Plato, *Symposium*, 58–60.

> It is not rude, it is not self-seeking,
> it is not easily angered, it keeps no record of wrongs.
> Love does not delight in evil but rejoices with the truth.
> It always protects, always trusts,
> always hopes, always perseveres (1 Cor 13:4–7).
>
> For I am convinced that neither death nor life,
> neither angels nor demons,
> neither the present nor the future, nor any powers,
> neither height nor depth, nor anything else in all creation,
> will be able to separate us from the love of God (Rom 8:38–39).

With little more than that, the Symposium began. Storm Swain was the first to speak. She suggested that I put up the opening slide, which was am image of Rafael's *School of Athens*.

She said, "So I begin with a confession that for me seems somewhat apropos. Six years ago, I was sitting in a prenatal class at Roosevelt Hospital in New York city, a forty-year-old woman, pregnant for the first time, watching a much older woman show us a technique, and show us as women and men, and women and women, a technique to get us through the hours of childbirth. This one particular technique the woman was showing us—I thought—was frankly pretty ridiculous. And I turned to my husband and said, 'You've got to be kidding, I'm never doing that.'

"Well, I have learned to say neither to God, nor a US Immigration official, 'You've got to be kidding.' But I'm thinking that maybe I should add midwives to that very short list.

"Like the rejected stone, this very silly—what seems like a silly—little technique, short breaths followed by 4, 5, 6, 5, 4 rhythm, [demonstration] and so on, followed by one long [demonstration] breath, got me through seventeen and one-half hours of labor [audible response of moans and groans from audience], before an emergency C-section.

"So such an experience gives me a window into the question of spiritual midwifery, and as a woman provides a challenge for me to some of the earlier comments in Stephen Faller's manuscript. At times it provides not just a challenge but a barrier, but also it was a place that I needed to get to see deeper into the heart of the subject.

"So the pastoral theologian Carrie Doehring suggests that in any pastoral endeavor we need to begin with self-reflection to see whether our own experience may be a resource or a roadblock in meeting the other. As

The Symposium

a woman, along with many of my colleagues, our first window into this material may well be—whether we are child-endowed, childless, or child free—the metaphor of midwifery through the lens initially of the birthing mother, and we may test the metaphor initially from the place of that reception rather than from identification of the midwife as our first movement. So as a woman I cannot listen to Socrates's claims to be a spiritual midwife, without a connection first to the reality of what midwives do and for whom they do it for. The metaphor for me needs us to move into that reality and out again, perhaps approaching and then retreating as we go forward. For me, such a movement is a deeply embodied place. It is an ensouled place. It is the place where we stand, or lie, or squat, depending on what practice we may follow in birthing. And like Stephen's own description of being at the birth of your first child and hearing today about the very quick birth of your second child, and on Karen Hansen's reflection on being a spiritual midwife at the labor and delivery of a child that she baptized as it took its first and last breath, that's the reality for where the metaphor comes from, from where I need to begin.

"It's the place that says the metaphor needs to be true to the reality, to include the messy reality of birth, not the cleaned up, idealized version, but the reality of sweat, blood, and tears. And it also needs to include the reality of death. Stephen's reflections on death and its relation to the authenticity of the dialogue of the soul, through the death of Socrates and Jesus, I think can take us to this place. And here we know that death is not the worst thing that can happen. But perhaps its here also that the metaphor may yet take us deeper into those baptismal resonances that we have in the spiritual life. And having been involved in hospital chaplaincy for about a decade, I know, as many of us do who have been called in those wee hours of the night to the maternity unit, that death of a child is as real a possibility as part of the birthing process as is the birth of a live child. And also we are reminded of the death of the mother also. So I confess, and whether theologically appropriate or not, I have baptized more dying and dead children than I would have liked to. Birth can be hard. The spiritual life can be hard. And being alongside another in this travail can also be hard.

"So, let me reflect on some moments in the manuscript in this hard, messy, sacred journey and see how the metaphor carries us, or carries me, and the understanding of birthing from this place.

"I'd like to connect the metaphor of midwifery to the birthing not only of the child but also the birthing of creation, on both a cosmic level and an interpersonal level. What gets created and I think Stephen was teasing out is a relational space. And for me Donald Winnicott speaks of this space very well. He speaks of the 'space-holding' and also the 'space-affording' mother and the ability of the mother to be alone with the child or 'alone in the presence of another'. And in some of your descriptions, Stephen, of the midwife and her role or his role, I think that speaks to the place that speaks to the ministry of presence and absence, the move . . . the approaching and the retreating. And I think also again about those liturgical absences that might also resonate the space of Holy Saturday and that wonderful liturgical space that comes after ascension and before Pentecost.

"But it is into the embodied space that I kept on looking for in the metaphor. And the focus on rhetoric at times felt like it negated the essential embodiment of the process. And yet one has to remember that it is not the midwife who is embodying the birthing and that doesn't need not to get lost. Otherwise I think if the sense of embodiment is lost. For me it can feel like a patriarchal appropriation of a woman's metaphor without attention to the woman's bodies it attends to. So perhaps more of a dialogue could lead me deeper into the metaphor to be able to work with the rhetoric in a different way.

"And I'm not suggesting this you have not done that, Stephen, but at times I looked for that in a way, and I thought it's something that seems particularly critical in this moment because that process is going on in the political sphere, an appropriation of women's bodies without women being part of the dialogue. So there is a need to somehow hold that in creative tension.

"So, at times, despite the focus on rhetoric to the extent that I began to fear the loss of embodiment, I want to say how taken I was again by the diaLogos play.

"And this description of dialogue with the Heraclitan origins of logos described for me so well actually not the moment of pastoral care but the preaching moment. And it took me back to remembering being at the cathedral of St. John the Divine and preaching there, which I did for about seven years. People would say to me, you know 'Why would you want to preach from such a high pulpit, so far away, so distant from the people, it's so removed?' And I have to tell you in that space it felt like an incredibly intimate dialogue. So there's something about intimate dialogue with a community that you know well, whether there is only one person doing the speaking or not, that it's not about geographical space, because I am

The Symposium

one of those people who hate supply preaching to a community that I don't know, even if the pulpit is really close to the people, or I'm in the middle of them. It's in that space with the unknown that it seems like the distance is greatest to me. It feels like a one-way communication that speaks more of a relational distance than my body being distant from those that I am in relationship with.

"So it's in this tension of otherness in such a dialogue ensues. What the midwife metaphor does offer in the way you've articulated it, even though I can get lost in the other pastoral metaphors, is the sense of alterity, the sense of Otherness, the focus on the other, not to the exclusion of the self but the focus on the other as the sense of authority—and that's where the metaphor grabbed me most. The midwife listens to the other and in so doing encourages the other to listen to the self. In pastoral metaphors that so often get caricatured or solidified, like the solicitous and courageous shepherd, that often encourage seminarians to think that they are to care for those that are somehow lesser than themselves, to dispense wise advice, and put that them in the anxiety-producing position of thinking that they need to be the ones who know what to do. I think the Socratic attitude that you're inviting us into offers both a brutally offensive counter to that and a gentle invitation to another way.

"As Stephen points out, what also needs not to get lost in the diaLogue is the sense of what is being born to the other also.

"In childbirth the fetus is not simply the other, as in a two-person dialogue, it is the third. There is something about a mystery of otherness for the one giving birth that can elude both the bearer and the midwife. In spiritual midwifery are we giving birth to that which is other, or that which is the self, or is the other the self, the true self that is other to the compliant social self, or the ego? What is being born? Or is it, as Jesus says, rebirth, the image of God perhaps being reborn in us in each relationship, God continually coming to life in our lives?

"Again, where the metaphor does grab me is the attention to movement. Margaret Kornfeld, whose metaphor is the Pastoral Careras Gardener, notes, we tend, we nurture, we cultivate, but God gives the growth. Like Kornfeld's miracle question has the follow-up, "How is that happening just a little bit already?" The focus is on the growth—the growth and the other.

"I was once in a psychodrama training workshop where we were doing some kind of role play. And this was early on in my ministry and I was using all my best attending, following, and reflective listening skills, and to do what? The brutally attentive psychodrama coach, who was a little too famous for his own good, said that what I was doing was bringing the person to a full-stop. His simple bit of direction that was transforming in the moment and has somewhat haunted me for years afterwards was, 'Go with the movement.' Stephen's attitude to this in both the individual and the group setting speaks well to the ability of the metaphor to live in communal settings, where we often question what it is to be pastoral. Go with the movement.

"So in the end I want to pick up this question of diaLogos, resonant with the Socratic questioning of Jesus perhaps, by offering a model that I was given, which I think on one level is an illustration of the midwifery method even if not drawing on the metaphor. And I'm just going to do this very quickly . . .

"The oral tradition of this model comes from Joan Dalloway, who is a New Zealand CPE supervisor, psychoanalyst, and on the faculty for a psychoanalysis training program.

"Dalloway's model focuses on what she calls the three pastoral questions, questions that a pastoral caregiver might keep in mind in attending to the other. In brief, the first question is based on the question of God to Adam and Eve in the garden of Eden after they had eaten of the tree of the fruit of the knowledge of good and evil (Gen 3:9). God asked the question to Adam, 'Where are you?'

"'Where are you?' It's a curious question for an omnipotent God. It's an invitation for the person to tell their own story. Although one would suppose that an omniscient and omnipotent creator in the text knows where the man is, God still asks the question. There is respect for the other in telling his own story and taking responsibility for his own actions. And in pastoral care in this midwifery method, I think, we are invited to not think that we know the story of the other and act accordingly, but to show that same respectful invitation for the other to share his own story and for that to be the focus rather than our knowledge.

"The second question comes from John 5:6, to the man who has been paralyzed for thirty-eight years. When Jesus saw him lying there, and he knew he had been there for a long time, he said, 'Do you want to be made well?'

"'Do you want to be made well?'—the question of Jesus to the invalid man at the pool of Bethesda.

The Symposium

"Jesus hears the man's history of thirty-eight years of being an invalid. It had been the style of his life for almost four decades. And rather than simply healing him without a 'by your leave,'[2] he leaves the decision up to the man himself. In essence the question is 'Do you want to change?'

"The third pastoral question is based on the question of Jesus to blind Bartimaeus (Mark 10:51). He asks blind Bartimaeus, 'What do you want me to do for you?' Once again Jesus does not take the position of greater knowledge, but asks the recipient to define the parameters of his care. This model of care doesn't assume that all the resources are with the pastoral caregiver or with the midwife, but sees the other as having resources for himself and the ability to ask for those he doesn't have. Again, it's a listening to the wisdom in those we are caring for as the midwife does.

"Here the focus is on the one needing care, rather than the one doing the caring. It is both a ministry of presence that holds the relational space, and as Stephen's speaks about, a ministry of absence, that affords the other space. Respect and empowerment define the boundaries of pastorhood in this model. Here, responsibility is modeled in a way that neither rescues nor abandons.

"So I think for me whether its Dalloway's three pastoral questions or the broader questions offered by a Socratic midwifery method, there is a sense that what's most powerful for me—" [At this point there was a deafening thunderclap. It had been lightning and storming and this interruption seemed like divine punctuation. We laughed. Without missing a beat, Swain looked upward and said, "Thank you."]

Then she continued, "What is most powerful for me, is a sense of not knowing the answers. It seems to me that it is the attitude that is the offered by this model that is the greatest gift of the method for me—that profound humility that reframes all those models which focus on the pastoral caregiver, whether it's the solicitous and courageous shepherd, the intimate stranger, the wounded healer, or even the wonderfully negating wise fool. So for me, this will offer another model that will be added to my repertoire, as I live into and center myself in the mystery of being in the travail of teaching in that profoundly privileged place where I get to see what is born in the lives and ministries of my students. Thank you so much."

With that, Storm sat down. I was humbled by the care and thought she put into her remarks on my work. I wanted to acknowledge her words, but

---

2. The critique of the cripple who is healed by Jesus, then loses his livelihood, in the movie Monty Python's *Life of Brian*.

The Symposium

also keep the Symposium moving. I said, "I'll be very brief. As Heraclitus says, 'The lightning directs everything.' I'll say this here: Part of what I am fighting against is a tradition that has buried a way of working with people. That same tradition is also used for writing for male readers, another tradition that needs to be challenged, with this very project."

There was a lot that Storm brought to the conversation. So much of what she said rang true. I enjoyed her efforts to bring in the liturgical absences into awareness, and I loved her reflections on baptism. Baptism is at once a symbol of life and death, a sacrament I have administered, and it registers powerfully with me. I did not want to engraft so strong a Christian symbol onto midwifery, but I'm glad to see that it's something a Christian theologian could do with the project.

I've taken a lot of her suggestions to heart, but I disagree with her on the matter of death. Of course, death always belongs, but here in the metaphor the mother and baby are one. Not that both people cannot die, because that happens too, but this is about learning how to midwife. And Jesus and Socrates both died their deaths in the service of a larger project. If anything is modeled here, it is the death of the midwife, not the tragic pathos of infant loss. Karen Hanson also resonates with a lot of Storm's sentiments (as did Art Pressley). She says that the minister as midwife necessarily takes on five duties: being able to identify travail, to be experienced, to be person-centered, the naming in birth, and dealing with death when necessary.[3] As true as this is, there is a very real difference between birth and infant hospice or infant palliative care. This is the space to be extremely attentive to the living process, and being distracted by the theology of infant loss is not helpful.

I invited anyone to speak, either on a similar theme, or a completely different theme. Debbie was the next to speak. She rose. And she challenged me right away, just like a chaplain: "Stephen, I want to challenge you to rethink your understanding of negation, by recasting it within the theology of kenosis. Kenosis is the Greek word for 'emptying' that is used in Philippians 2:7. As you have referenced in your manuscript, Paul says, 'Christ poured himself out, taking the form of a servant.' In Christ's spiritual emptying I think we gain great insight in how we are called to be the spiritual midwife for others. While you have stated that the negation theory puts the midwife on the periphery of the central work of the conversation, kenosis theology

---

3. See Hanson, "The Midwife."

places the spiritual midwife at the center of the spiritual dynamic within the pastoral care conversation.

"As a chaplain I lived out this theological understanding of kenosis as a key part of my ministry of presence. Kent Groff describes the qualities of kenosis as willing surrender of one's ego-driven self and enmeshment in one's own issues in order to move into a God-centered contemplative mode when one enters a pastoral conversation. This is not negation of the person of the caregiver, but rather the invitation of the presence of the divine through the conduit of the person of the caregiver. The person of the caregiver is very much needed—used—by the divine in offering care that centers on the patient.

"Because we only speak briefly today let me use an example from my pastoral work to illustrate kenosis as a key element of pastoral care. As a chaplain, before I entered each room I would wash my hands and use these words to meditate during this time of cleansing: 'Clean hands, clean heart. Clean hands, clean heart.' During those brief moments I would release my cares and anxieties of the day, the concerns of other patients I had already seen, and my plans for the rest of the day, in order to enter a space where my spirit was open to listening to the patients and also to listen to how the divine was prompting me to respond. During the visit I would be myself, with all my special createdness, gifts, and flaws, but I would also always be attuned to listening for the depth of the issues that the patient was discussing, and seeking a place for the Holy to enter the room through our reflections together. Gentle patient-centered questions are sometimes a vital part of the visit. Using kenosis theology is not about employing special listening techniques. It is about using all one's excellent reflective listening skills, with an ear to the Holy rather than to one's own natural responses. As I would leave the room, I again would wash my hands, and meditate on the words, 'Clean hands, clean heart.' This would allow me to lift in prayer this particular visit and prepare me for the next person who I would meet on my journey.

"I would encourage you to explore the literature on the theology of kenosis, and embrace the theology of kenosis as part of the ministry of presence rather than positing 'negation and the ministry of absence as a complementary modality to the ministry of presence.'"

She sat down. I said, "Thank you. I'm so thankful that I have your remarks and that I can study and meditate on them. But I can ask you a question now: You're asking me to reconsider negation and this idea, the entire idea of the ministry of absence?"

She said, "Yeah. I have heard the ministry of absence coined, rather than being a real representation of what I think the ministry of presence encompasses by the theology of kenosis."

I replied, "Okay, interesting. And very helpful. Some of the things that Socrates did, for example using the midwifery as a male, was precisely for the 'pop,' that something had to shock, and I have apologized to my trainees on multiple occasions that I tend to speak in hyperbole, which may have led me to this language of the ministry of absence. Thank you for your heartfelt words and the experience of how God has been with you on your journey."

I have thought heavily about where Debbie confronted me. Some of the things I write because I believe they are universal. Some things I write because, as I learned from my Kierkegaard studies, sometimes a corrective is needed. Such things are not universal or dogmatically correct, but remain necessary for the time. I have also come to believe that some things are universally needed as a corrective. We always need to be reminded to repent.

I think that the "ministry of presence" is always going to be tricky and dangerous, in that we are ever tempted to understand that to meet our own ends. We are ever tempted to fuse the ministry of presence with self-affirmation. Furthermore, I think that there are negative forms of spirituality, *via negativa*, that are always elusive and hidden, because humans beings are always beguiled by the things that are there instead of the things that are not. Debbie speaks for the best of the "presence tradition"—what she spoke is true because she is true. She represents something important here and authentic. But I think that the highest forms of spirituality and self-sacrifice are always counterintuitive, and we need to remember to find them.

I do like what Fred Craddock says on the issue. He writes, "It is most difficult for the communicator to accept as a model the Incarnation, emptying oneself, making oneself of no reputation for the sake of others. The demanding point here is that it takes more than a Christian subject to have a Christian communication. Christ has given us the 'how' as well as the 'what.'"[4] I think this gets to the heart of it and it is something I've found compelling from the beginning. Spiritual midwifery was never intended to be a Christian concept strictly for Christian practitioners; however, I have always found it strange that so many Christians are completely unaware of

---

4. Craddock, *Overhearing the Gospel*, 54.

The Symposium

the way Jesus worked, virtually unaware of his style, as if it were heretic to suggest that he had style. Admittedly, it's easier said than done. Craddock also says, "I confess it is easier to try to master the 'what' than to be mastered by the 'how.'"[5]

Johann spoke next. She said with a transparent honesty, "I appreciate the opportunity to serve as reader of this book and am very impressed by this dialogical process of reviewing this manuscript. I mean, this is amazing—every book should be written this way. It's a great process. My strongest attraction to the book is the central metaphor of midwifery. So much of what you want this book to do is evoked by this powerful image. In particular, your desire to understand spiritual midwifery as that which assists, helps to bring forward and nurture in a natural, noninvasive way benefits from the allusion to actual midwifery. Your wish to decenter the pastoral minister and to emphasize the indirect ways in which this ministry ought to proceed are similarly brought to light by the use of this metaphor. The greatest attraction of the book for me is its emphasis on openness, agility, and flexibility. I appreciate its stated purpose to sketch the contours of an art, or a process, rather than pound out every detail of a procedure. Indeed for this end as well, the analogy with midwifery is particularly effective.

I am not versed in the theory or practice of pastoral care. My background is in Catholic systematic theology and parish ministry, particularly in the ministry of Christian formation. In both my writing and my teaching, I am lately quite occupied with the topic of formation—spiritual formation for a particular set of practices—for the Christian life in general, and in particular for solidarity with the suffering. So this book surfaced several connections for me. I believe its ideas, especially those of helping to bring forth what is about to be born spiritually in the other, are compatible with basic good practices in the ministries of catechesis, in preaching, and in spiritual direction, as we've said. The decentering of the minister and focus on the one who is laboring seems to me to be a needed corrective in any area of ministry. Further, the book led me to ask, what is the appropriate means of formation for spiritual midwifery in pastoral care? What are the practices, when engaged in repeatedly and with reflection, that can form in the pastoral care practitioner the necessary dispositions to engage in spiritual midwifery as you've described it?

"Now you've mentioned the word *mysticism*. And your question about where do you find the riches and the literature on care of the soul. And you

---

5. Ibid.

know, I think you're definitely going through the rhetorical and philosophical traditions, but it may be interesting to put that into dialogue with the mystical traditions or with traditions of spiritual formation. So I work with nuns, the Sisters of Mercy. And just in a meeting the other day the president of our university was talking about when she was a novice and the practices that she had to do every week and reporting to her spiritual director. Very practically speaking, these practices that have been used throughout the centuries in Christian traditions but also of course in other world religious traditions as well, to form in a person a certain spiritual disposition. So I just wonder if that's a resource also for this project.

"To what extent are the ideas and emphases presented in this book already a part of the formation process for pastoral care ministry? I don't know that, having never gone through CPE, so maybe you could tell me that. And to what extent do they still need to be incorporated? I think that would also be a fruitful area to pursue for this volume, or for a subsequent treatment, as you've said, both for the consideration of spiritual midwifery for pastoral care, as well as for the formation for this particular orientation to ministry in other fields."

I replied, "I have a lot to think about. Thank you all. You had a question . . ."

"To what extent is the formation for this practice done in CPE or chaplaincy?"

I said, "Recently I have shifted from chaplain to CPE supervisor, and there's a natural evolution that goes with the caring of souls of patients to the caring of souls of caregivers. In many ways for me it's an evolution that is not complete, but the way that you have framed your question has inspired within me a new interest in this. When it comes to the teaching of midwifery there is always this twin polarity that it's something I want to do and something I'm afraid of doing because chaplains come into the pastoral program to learn not about my interests but about themselves. But owning this pedagogical component will be a necessary part of my development."

Tim was the next up. He said, "I am honored to be included in this Symposium; to have the privilege of reading and reviewing Stephen's innovative manuscript on spiritual midwifery, and to add my reflections to those of the esteemed colleagues who are gathered here today.

"My training and practice is in practical ministry, my primary professional work for more than twenty years, and my work now as a marriage and family therapist, which is my current professional work for more than

The Symposium

ten years. I am a practitioner rather than a researcher or deep thinker, and I state that with a little bit of hesitation but also with a little bit of confidence because that's who I am and that's where I want to be. ["Amens" abound from the audience.] My studies in the disciplines of theology and philosophy enabled me both to graduate from seminary and be an effective pastor. However, I do not claim to be well read or an 'expert' in either of these fields. But most of my studies over the past twenty years have been in the area of systems theory, with application both toward pastoral ministry and psychotherapy.[6] Some of those who have bridged that use of systems theory, which started in the family and has also expanded to organizations like the church with Mia Friedman, Peter Steinke (one of my favorites), and Ron Richardson, coming out of the Lutheran tradition. In addition, I am privileged to teach students preparing for pastoral ministry, chaplaincy, and pastoral counseling at Palmer Theological Seminary. I value the challenge to integrate my pastoral and psychological learning and to try to impart that or to instill a hunger in the students to be able to make that integration as well between pastoral theology and psychological practice.

"My contribution to this Symposium, Steve, is a recommendation to include concepts of systems theory in the work you've done on spiritual midwifery. I do not see this inclusion as raising a conflicting voice, but rather one that will deepen your insights and integration of spirituality and philosophy together with the field of psychology. The common thread that ties these disciplines together is that of the importance of relationships.

"In chapter 2 of your manuscript the primacy of relationships takes center stage as you define dialogue. This relational activity is much more than two (or more) people interacting through words. But rather through the experience of dialogue there is the defining of the 'I' and the 'Thou' (to use Buber's concepts). Systems theorists see a clear parallel to this defining an 'I' and a 'Thou' in Murray Bowen's seminal work on family systems theory, specifically the concept of differentiation. Interpersonal differentiation describes the creative tension between two primary needs that we all have: the need to identify with community and the need to be identified as an individual. The well-differentiated person, and the well differentiated relationship, encourages all participants—so in this case both the one who is seeking spiritual growth and transformation and the spiritual midwife—to claim both of these identities, part of the community and that of individual,

---

6. System theory was first applied to families, and then to congregational systems through the innovative work of Friedman, Steinke, and Richardson.

without sacrificing either. Your description of effective dialogue, which I found most effectively contained in your caution about the cost of political correctness, is a plea to avoid achieving inclusivity by sacrificing identity. I would also point out the error of the 'other' to achieve identity by sacrificing inclusivity. To paraphrase the words of my first clinical supervisor, a healthy relationship is one in which there is 'room to be me, room to be you, and room to be us.' Spiritual midwifery encourages the development of such space, and trusts in the maturing outcome of both parties.

"Other systems theory concepts that could provide at least additional terminology and perhaps significantly greater depth are tied to your chapters on 'Indirect Communication,' 'Negation,' and the importance of movement in 'Inductive Logic.' I will briefly make these connections tonight within the time constraints of this Symposium, and anticipate opportunities to continue this discussion in the future.

"Concepts of 'indirect communication' identify the importance of content and process—what systems theorists and practitioners call 'metacommunication.' This level of interaction is communication at the deeper, relational level. Spiritual growth occurs when the communications between spiritual seeker and spiritual midwife, between spiritual seeker and God, and between spiritual midwife and God, operate effectively to connect—or to say it in other words, the content is what we're talking about. The process or metacommunication is how we're talking about that and what that says about our relationship.

"Your description of negation can also be explained in systems terms as complementary relationships. 'Complementary' not in the sense of 'that's an attractive outfit' or 'your hair looks nice today' but complementary in the sense that one person's actions and activity define or help to define the behavior of another person and vice versa. When the effective spiritual midwife steps back to allow space for growth, this practice can be described as using overfunctioning and underfunctioning terminology. Just as a leader needs followers in order to maintain his/her role, so pastoral counselors, chaplains, and therapists who insert themselves too much into the process will 'train' others to be dependent. This overfunctioning, usually unintentional and certainly unconscious, defines the role of the spiritual seeker to accept a 'one down' role in his functioning rather than one of growth. The potential for spiritual birth and spiritual growth when this happens is stunted.

The Symposium

One final word about systems theory and indirect logic. You define deductive logic as causal and inductive logic as predictive, which then defines the learning process and the relationship. I would encourage also use of the term *circular thinking*, where each person in the exchange is both influenced by the actions of another and influencing the other by her own actions. I would encourage this as a third interconnected model, where the learning and growth affects everyone involved in the process. In working with couples or with families I often will look at what's the relational dance, what's the family dance. What am I doing that's influencing you, and what are you doing that's influencing me, and I'm intrigued to see how that can happen, does happen, could happen in the idea of spiritual transformation and spiritual midwifery.

Again, thank you for this invitation and opportunity to learn together. Speaking only for myself, you have succeeded."

I replied, "Thank you." The warmth of his words stunned me into a moment of silence. After thinking, I added, "There is a lot to what you said. And something at the very beginning struck me as extremely profound, with the differentiation between the self and the other. I think that however popular Buddhism and atheism become, one thing that we monotheists will always have going for us is the sense that there is a Creator, and we are not it. That there is this essential awareness of self and other that we explore in the fabric of reality, and perhaps that is always the primal and primary relationship upon which other relationships are based. So, wonderful stuff. I am thankful for your remarks, and the time you spent with my project."

The evening moved on. The clinking of forks, knives, and china started to slow, as did the rain from the thunderstorm. With a big smile, Willard Ashley stood up. "Confession is good for the soul. Growing up a good Catholic, confession was part of my regular routine along with fish on Fridays. Today I have a confession. I hear voices!

"Before you reach for the DSM-IV of V or pick up the phone to make a referral, hear me out. Reading the manuscript was moved down on my list of things to do. NBTS granted me tenure and less than eighteen hours after learning of the report of the tenure review committee our president asked me to serve as Acting Dean of the Seminary. My world has been turned upside down, complete with various voices. The voices are of students asking for a change of grade. The voices are of faculty colleagues working to design a new curriculum. The voices are of my choir members singing the Lord's song even under the most dire of circumstances. The voices are of my

The Symposium

patients who ask, 'So, doc is this normal?' (And we go, 'Define normal?') The voices are of my wife, who says, 'Honey I am so proud of you. Now here is your Honey Do list. And by the way, the grass looks a little long in the yard.' The voices are of my body that reminds of my age. The voices are of my son, who called to say, 'Dad! The Heat win! NBA champs!' The voices are of my editor, who reminds me that my edits for my next book are due in two weeks. There I sit looking at my downloaded copy of your manuscript while all the realities of real life sink into my head. It is here, at this place, at this point, where your manuscript, Stephen, demanded my attention and did not allow me to put it down until I had finished reading it.

"Your manuscript is excellent in so many ways; but not perfect, yet. Reading it gave me answers to questions not asked out loud. It gave me peace and comfort. In my new role, the manuscript in its unfinished state will serve me well. Okay, so much for the narcissistic ramblings. Others will find this book to be a good guide to leadings others be it in medicine, law, education, ethics, or economics.

"Your manuscript challenges, confronts and comforts as does Benjamin Valentin, *In Our Own Voices*;, as does Joel LeMon, *Method Matters*; as does Carmen Nanko-Fernandez, *Theologizing en Espanglish*; and as does Randel Jelks, *Benjamin Elijah Mays: School Master of the Movement*. Your work is intellectual, passionate, and begs for critical reflection. Thank you!

"As we look at the work, my general reaction to the project was one of delight that Stephen tackled the subject and trepidation as to how his project will be received in a growing anti-intellectual climate. We live in an information age, whereby people digest mountains of data without any or seemingly little critical reflection as to the source of the information along with the history and agenda of the writers. Can spiritual midwifery engage in a conversation that is intellectual, contextual, and culturally competent? Will Stephen's project accomplish his stated goals? Will the written pages deliver what he advertises or will I leave the pages still seeking to understand/apply the concept of spiritual midwifery?

"The logic of the project made sense. The chapters demonstrated a logical flow. I am not sure that the chapter titles are 'sexy' enough or alluring to the reader at first glance. Chapter titles inform and invite. Perhaps some strengthening of the wording of the chapter titles is needed or least revising the titles in terms of book sales. People read the table of contents to make a decision to buy the book and unless you are a famous author

The Symposium

or selling sex as in *Fifty Shades of Grey*, you will need a table of contents that pulls the reader in.

"The greatest strength of the manuscript was Stephen's use of the metaphor and his smooth way of helping the reader to understand why this is important in one's work and life. Whereby the chapter headings did not draw me in clearly his content did draw me into his work. I love the concept of the quotes at the start of each chapter and the summary at the end of each chapter. My students will read the quote and the summary and call it a day! We can talk about quote selection later.

"The manuscript has a strange twist to it. The title talks of spiritual midwifery, however many of the 'scholarly' quotes are from men. Women are guides in delivery; however, their voices seem silent in other places in the book. Women have an implied leadership role in the book that is perhaps not as demonstrative as the men.

"It is with hesitancy that I lift this up, but in my circles the philosophers quoted borrowed their thinking from black scholars without the benefit of acknowledgement. You want to research this and give it mention. To this end, you may want to broaden your perspective to include thinking/ theology from the 1040 corridor and seek intentionality in giving women a scholarly voice in the book.

"The book possesses great potential. Again, Stephen, I am delighted that you are taking on this subject matter and I enjoy your treatment of it. The book can and will make a contribution to pastoral care. Clearly, the book can actually be a guide for mentors, CPE supervisors, field educators, practical theologians, teachers, and even parents. It is both intellectual and practical.

"Allow me to suggest that you do not limit the book to pastoral care. It can also serve as a text for leadership development. If you add some illustrations (drawings to be exact) you can probably market the book to parents. You can pitch the book to business executives, particularly executive coaches. Much of the wisdom of the book is Coaching 101. You may consider a second book that is the popular shorter version for the Barnes & Noble crowd: *Coaching 101: Wisdom from Midwives*. Teachers of theology may make use of the book. It again can be used for field education.

"As I mentioned before, your bibliography is almost if not totally exclusively men. It weakens an excellent work.

The Symposium

"You are on to something of significance. We can explore in person what question your book raises, who is asking the question and does it matter (Max Stackhouse 101)?

"Thus allow me to conclude with a few more questions. Why did you really write the book? And the therapist's question, why now? What really drove you to write this book? Who is your intended audience? Will you include a DVD or link to a web page? Are you ready for the book to change your life as it will change the lives of others? Thank you! Thank you for allowing us to journey with you in this endeavor. May we be your midwives in this project."

I was overwhelmed by all the feedback. I began to respond, "So I think about the dialogues of Plato where there's this discussion and someone says something brilliant and Socrates takes it in, digests it, and adds to it. Or the Gospels where Jesus is in dialogue and says exactly the right thing without repeating. How did they do that?"

Will had some important objections. I continued, "One thing is for sure: the book needs to do more with women's voices. I don't know if I can find the female perspective on the Socratic irony that I want but I am not limited to that. I work with midwives and several have mentioned female philosophers, scholars, and teachers that I might refer to. So we'll see what's there.

"This has been an ongoing challenge in the project. There are not a lot of sources, male for female, that look at Socratic irony as it relates to spiritual midwifery. But I look at those who have employed the midwifery, and those who named it, and offer both."

With a smile, I went on, "As to the sexiness of the chapter titles . . . the Tao says, 'Beautiful words are not true, and true words are not Beautiful.' However, Diotima, who we started with, has something to say about the nature of beauty and truth together. People have to be inspired from afar to come forth and engage this project, so I think there's something there that can make it stronger, because if this is going to be life-giving there needs to be some sexiness about it, that's what life is all about."

Art Pressley stood up next. He has a soft-spoken nature, which magnifies the philosophical and ethical tone to his words. He couples this with a folksy philosophical style. He said, "Just a couple of comments, as I've given a lot of my reflection throughout the day. When I read the book I was very excited about it. I wanted to pass it out to my students so I could have conversations about it. There was something about it. I think we talked about that?"

"Yes," I agreed we had talked about that.

He went on, "But there was something distressing about it. I've been struggling with it since I read it. And part of it could be simply that I have a wacky mind. That's true.

"The other part, I started out my ministry clinical work as part of a trauma unit. It was at a hospital on the south side of Chicago, and I worked there as a chaplain on the trauma team. And what I noticed about myself after my first year was that I had no problem with a lot of the trauma, be it an airplane crash, train wrecks, shootings (we were close to the housing projects)—regardless of what came through the door as chaplain or minister I had no problem, but when women were about to give birth they couldn't find me. Childbirth they couldn't get me near. And that's a part of the reason I struggle with the term *midwife*. There's a part of the term that almost suggests that this is a normal healthy process that people need to be respectful of as they're standing outside of. And most of our babies ended up in neonatal care. So understanding the role of the midwife when you don't have this normal, healthy, almost romanticized process of moving toward this new identity after suffering, but you're having something where it is far more complex than that because as many babies were not making it as were making it. And so I'm understanding that you're talking about midwife as this metaphor the way we're connecting metaphor to those groundings of life, but I struggled with it.

"This moves me to my next question. When I was starting seminary the big term was the feminization of ministry. And I guess that's why I raise this question about being engendered. When they were talking about the feminization of ministry, this is not something that people were celebrating. When people talked about feminization they were talking about gender constructs relating to any part of life—particularly for the men in the room talking about feminization of ministry—and they were depressed. What they meant was loss of control of one's life, loss of power and status. There was an expectation that ministers were to be more passive, there was almost a masochistic quality.

"As we're using the term for the larger culture, I'm not certain how we feel about it as a culture. I like the idea of the spiritual midwife, but I would want to complexify a bit it in a way that is also consistent with these births that don't come to life, or loss of status, or what it means to participate in

The Symposium

healing when there is this assumption that women's way of being in relationship may be very different than your classical Greek way of being in relationship. Which may be closer to alterity—and Winnicott's surviving object...."

Art was taking the dialogue in an important direction. At some level, I am guilty of exploring the limits of language, and I'm trying to explore this idea of midwifery with some precision. But how people really connect doesn't rely on language. Women may have very different ways of being and connecting in the world that have nothing to do with what Socrates and Kierkegaard have done with irony. Fair. And we should be careful of superimposing language that excludes other ways of being. Also fair.

We may find ourselves in relationships with those who have had identities imposed on them—perhaps even imposed on our language of relationship. Art argued for a position that hoped for something "more intersubjective and interdependent." And he furthered, "There may be multiple ways of connecting. And depending on how you're understanding classical philosophical tradition, if it's also Du Bois and Baldwin, etc., or only Kierkegaard and Tillich."

For me, it has never been a question of who owns the metaphor of midwifery, or even spiritual midwifery. Hindu thought probably had it first. And it has never been a question of which scholars belong at the table; by definition, all of them do. But rather, if there is a way of working with the soul—through dialogue—embedded right in the heart of the Jesus and Socrates movements, as Girard likes to say, "things hidden since the foundation of the world," what is that way?

"Just one other thing," Art remarked. "I really like your negation. It reminds me of apophatic theology, when it's understood that identity, close to Shelly Rambo, assumes that that which cannot be spoken, is where God truly is. Even if you can't name it, there is a presence but it is in the void that respects who we are and that honors that which was lost. There new identities can come forth. Thank you."

I really enjoyed Art's remarks. I offered, "I see the need for addressing the reality that death happens, but while this approach to pastoral care may be wonderful and life-giving, it is not without peril."

Debbie rejoined the conversation, "Spiritual midwife was only a positive concept for me as having three healthy children. Now that I have listened to several other people talking about this, I am really rethinking the term as it is no longer romanticized. "

The Symposium

I nodded, "I think it is helpful. Plato is nothing without his idealization. That's not where we live. In future research I'll want to do more with the apophatic, and also the Greek concept of *aporia*, the great not-knowing. Every trainee is confronted with the unknown, where there is nothing to say."

But I was also convicted by some of Art's other challenges, especially with Du Bois and Baldwin but also Toni Morrison. I think a risk in a project like mine is accidently marginalizing other thinkers when I'm trying so very hard to give voice to ideas that I believe have been marginalized. The standard guard against this is to detail how spiritual midwifery fits into the nexus of philosophy itself. Where do these ideas come from? Who has touched them?

To be sure, there is a prehistory of spiritual midwifery. Just as Socrates confidently illustrates his points with Greek mythology, we would be well-served to go back to their contextual Egyptian narrative. And equally sure, the philosophy of dialectic is certainly not limited to Socrates and his contemporary dialecticians. But to really elaborate how spiritual midwifery fits into the fabric of human thought would really require a different focus than my own: what is this spiritual midwifery of Jesus and Socrates?

Another academic question lies in the church: how has the church understood spiritual rebirth across the centuries? How has it understood the history of helping and enabling that rebirth? Again, these are interesting questions, but not here.

Barbara was the last to speak. She made her way to the front, with all sorts of books with her. With poise, she began, "I'm not trained in any of these fields, pastoral counseling or philosophy. I am an unreformed English major, and a writer. And a person for whom words and transformation that words can bring. Poets and poems have been midwives to me."

She then cleared her throat and titled her work, "The Grammar of Poetry." And then, "Prelude."

"Attunement. Stephen, you began your manuscript with a description of the tuning of a symphony orchestra, a sound recognized by many. You likened it to a spiritual struggle for attunement, a search for balance. A listening.

"I agree. Last evening I heard the Philadelphia Orchestra play Dvorak and Rimsky-Korsakov. As the orchestra tuned hidden behind a large screen, the audience quieted, waiting, poised, imagining the beauty to come. The tuning was like an invitation. We all accepted.

The Symposium

"Your manuscript is an invitation to imagine a new grammar for the spiritual connection between people and with God, especially in the pastoral care setting, but I think not limited to that. You begin with the power of metaphor and language itself to help form that connection, choosing the central metaphor of midwifery.

"The idea that most intrigues me is not that metaphor itself, but the very use of metaphor and other figurative language as essential for this journey toward transformation. It is as if the language itself, in the dialectical conversations between two, offers a guide for the journey Godward.

"I think this is a language borrowed from the poet. And the importance of language itself, of Word, you ground in the ancient Greek use of logos, as introduced by Heraclitus and mirrored in Genesis in God's creative speaking the world into being, and in John's Gospel, where Jesus himself is Word of God. Bravo!

"The language of poetry, I posit, adheres to many of the concepts you outline. Poetic language takes metaphor and other figures of speech (alliteration, onomatopoeia, assonance, etc.) as its grammar. (See your chapter 1.) And as you point out, the Jesus statement, "The kingdom of God is like . . ." chooses metaphor as the grammar of that quality of love and community that will transform us all and all the world.

"The language of poetry is a dialogue, albeit one dialogue partner is usually silent (the reader/hearer). (Could this relate to your idea of a ministry of absence? And what about pastoral care conversations with people who cannot speak, for one reason or another, and are silent partners?) The poet offers, through words and images and silences/pauses, an invitation to see the world a certain way, and to see oneself in a certain light, and the reader/hearer responds. There is deep listening in poetry, as in the role of the midwife. There is also movement (dynamic) as you describe in your chapter 2.

"The language of poetry represents indirect communication (your chapter 3). The grammar of the poet does not deal in objectivity or facts. I like what you say in this chapter about Kierkegaard's contributions to understanding subjective versus objective. 'The Socratic secret, which can be infinitized in Christianity . . . is that movement inward, that truth of a subject's transformation within himself' and 'the *how* of the truth is precisely the truth.'

"And of course irony is part of poetry's grammar. Kierkegaard urges us (you say) to think about the relationship between form and content,

The Symposium

between inner and outer reality. These are the questions of the poet, the stuff of poems.

"There is so much more to say about the language of poetry and how I believe it mirrors much of what you are saying about the metaphor of the midwife in the journey to birth/rebirth and transformation. But to some poems!

"Poetry/midwifery offers material about movement, dynamic journeying, and the 'Way.' It is not about the destination, but about the way. It reminds me of Walt Whitman's 'Song of the Open Road.'

"And, along the lines of journeying, there is the wonderful movie, *The Way*, that Martin Sheen stars in, about a man whose son has died while traveling the Camino Santiago (the Way of St. James) in France and Spain, and who himself decides to take the Way. In the 'how' of the journey, he meets the unexpected companions who 'midwife' his rebirth.

"Walt Whitman also has a lovely poem about the soul that I think would support/illustrate your chapter on the soul. It is titled 'A Noiseless Patient Spider.'

"Then there is the poem by David Whyte titled 'Faith.'

"And his poem 'The Well of Grief.'

"Or Mary Oliver's 'The Summer Day,' which asks the essentially theological question 'Who made the world?' (Though as you say, Stephen, asking questions can be a dangerous pastoral care strategy!)

"Or Alice Walker's poems 'We Alone' and 'Expect Nothing.'

"Speaking of Alice Walker, the title of one of her volumes of poetry is *Horses Make a Landscape Look More Beautiful*. The title and the book's epigraph comes from a Native American shaman who wrote this about the violent intrusion of white settlers into Indian land: 'We can forgive you for bringing us guns and whiskey because you gave us the horse, *sunkawattan*, holy dog. And horses make the landscape more beautiful.'[7]

"The saying connects, I think, with your story about Roberts's horse whispering in the application chapter. It is about respect, and about equality, and about transformation.

"Getting back to grammar/syntax, and your comments on the connections of form and content. I noticed that your writing style throughout the manuscript was mainly subject-verb-object. Sentence after sentence followed this very direct communication pattern. Subject-verb-object. I wonder how your focus on indirect communication might influence a

---

7. Walker, *Horses Make a Landscape Look More Beautiful*.

writer's style. How do style and grammar of your sentence structure relate to your comments about form following content, or not?

"Do I have time for a few words about pedagogy that your paper raises for me? How do seminaries teach midwifery? How do students who will be ministers and pastoral counselors learn the role? Per your comments, today's students have a lot more opportunity to understand the mind of psychology than the mystical spirituality of medieval Christianity. That is certainly true at Princeton Seminary. How might classroom education and field education address this imbalance or lack? Who will be the teachers?

"And in the context of today's major focus on measurable assessment and outcomes/results in seminary education, how does that fit with your thinking in this manuscript? It seems counter to the philosophical ideas and commitments you discuss. Can you address this? Of course the same focus on assessment and measurable outcomes characterizes the church today: How many members do we have? How many attend worship and programs? How many children do we have in the Sunday school? Your book would suggest other, more pertinent questions: How are lives transformed through this church? How do we companion each other, guide one another toward God?

"I agree wholeheartedly with, and have experienced myself, the ineffectiveness and discomfort of pastoral care (especially in hospital) that is too determinative, too declarative, too focused on the caregiver, and on the caregiver 'doing something' or saying the 'right' prayer or 'being a ministry of presence,' that now sacralized and totemic phrase of which we may not know the meaning (as you address in your manuscript).

"I think overall that your approach to pastoral care using the metaphor of midwifery is full of potential for effective transformative relationships in the aura of who Jesus is and who he calls us to be. I think the manuscript would benefit from the addition of 'poetic grammar': examples from the poets and their poems. Poets, like midwives and the philosophers you cite, and Jesus himself, tend to come at things from the side.

"Can I end with two personal examples? I am not a hospital chaplain or a full-time pastor. But I can relate one experience where I believe I was a midwife. It was on a sailboat in Greece with a group of friends, all of whom had attended church as children, but none of whom was then part of a faith community. We visited Delphi, and saw the place of the Oracle of Delphi, to which you referred. That night, back on the boat, I don't know what strange spirit possessed me, but I dressed in scarves and beads, lit candles in my

The Symposium

small cabin, and invited each friend to come talk with the Oracle. I waited, silent. Then they came, one by one. Laughing, not sure if I was serious. And we talked about their lives, some fear, or hope, I can't remember the details. When the time was right, they stood and left the cabin. Something significant had been born. Each of the eight sailors came, one by one. Laughter, irony, image, silence, dialogue, the moments were poetry, really, where things were not as expected, and words opened up new worlds.

"This morning, as I prepared to come here, I sat on my deck reviewing my thoughts. A mourning dove flew to the deck, as often happens. I thought of my mother, who in her grief right after my father's death, saw and heard a mourning dove on the telephone pole near her house, and it comforted her. Whenever she saw and heard a dove thereafter, she thought of Dad and was comforted. Mourning dove. Bird of our grief. Or, morning dove, bird of our new beginnings."

Barbara was finished. I answered, "Your words have touched me deeply. We know Peter and others fished before they were called by Jesus, and Plato was a poet before called by Socrates. So maybe there is a mandate to do something poetic.

"Another way your words touch me is that in 2005 I was being awarded certification as a board certified chaplain. I had already begun this midwifery journey, and I thought, 'Am I on the right path? Was this some academic obsession?' Richard Rohr, who is a wonderful speaker, was talking about this great kind of dialectic and breaking open of liminal space where people are forced into situations they can't control. And I took it as a confirmation of my path as a vocation. And he read a poem by an author you mentioned, David Whyte. It feels like it's come full circle.

"It's been a long day. I want to thank you all for coming." And with little more than that, we gathered things together, with a very warm goodbye, and headed out into the summer night.

I think what surprised me was the feeling of it. Our recreation of Plato's symposium actually became a symposium. It wasn't a conference with an agenda, after which we dragged ourselves home. But like any of Plato's dialogues, our words had been true. We had found, through relationship and dialogue, a kind of rhetorical transcendence. Heraclitus says, "After death comes nothing—either hoped for or imagined."[8] And for my part, what we had created was better than anything I had hoped for.

---

8. Heraclitus, *Fragments*, 83.

Bibliography

Allen, Diogenes. *Philosophy for Understanding Theology*. Atlanta: John Knox, 1985.
Anderson, Herbert. "The Recovery of Soul." In *Treasure of Earthen Vessels*, edited by Brian Childs and David Waanders, 208–23. Louisville: Westminster John Knox, 1989.
Bogia, B. Preston. "Responding to Questions in Pastoral Care." *Journal of Pastoral Care* 39, no. 4 (1985) 357–69.
Brickhouse, T. C., and Nicholas D. Smith. *The Trial and Execution of Socrates: Sources and Controversies*. New York: Oxford University Press, 2002.
Craddock, Fred. *Overhearing the Gospel: Preaching and Teaching the Faith to Persons Who Have Already Heard*. Nashville: Abingdon, 1978.
Crossan, John Dominic. *The Dark Interval*. Sonoma, CA: Polebridge, 1988.
Frankl, Victor. *The Doctor and the Soul*. Translated by Richard and Clara Winston. New York: Vintage, 1986.
Geldard, Richard. *Anaxagoras and Universal Mind*. New York: Ralph Waldo Emerson Institute, 2007.
———. *Remembering Heraclitus*. Hudson, NY: Lindisfarne, 2000.
Gill-Austern, Brita L. "The Midwife, Storyteller, and Reticent Outlaw." In *Images of Pastoral Care: Classic Readings*, edited by Robert Dykstra, 218–27. St. Louis: Chalice, 2005.
Gordon, Jill. "Against Vlastos on Complex Irony." *The Classical Quarterly*, New Series, 46 (1996) 131–37.
Gottlieb, Paula. "The Complexity of Socratic Irony: A Note on Professor Vlastos." *The Classical Quarterly*, New Series, 42 (1992) 278–79.
Gouwens, David J. *Kierkegaard as Religious Thinker*. New York: Cambridge University Press, 1996.
Guenther, Margaret. *Holy Listening: The Art of Spiritual Direction*. Kindle ed. Lanham, MD: Rowman and Littlefield, 1992.
Hanson, Karen R. "The Midwife." In *Images of Pastoral Care: Classic Readings*, edited by Robert Dykstra, 249–56. St. Louis: Chalice, 2005.
Heraclitus. *Fragments: The Collected Wisdom of Heraclitus*. Translated by Brooks Haxton. New York: Viking, 2001.
Jaspers, Karl. *Anaximander, Heraclitus, Parmenides, Plotinus, Laotzu, Nagarjuna*. Edited by Hannah Arendt. Translated by Ralph Manheim. New York: Harcourt, 1990.
———. *Socrates, Buddha, Confucius, Jesus*. Edited by Hannah Arendt. Translated by Ralph Manheim. New York: Harcourt, 1990.

Bibliography

Kierkegaard, Søren. *The Concept of Irony with Continual Reference to Socrates.* Edited and translated by Howard V. Hong and Edna H. Hong. Princeton, NJ: Princeton University Press, 1989.

———. *Concluding Unscientific Postscript to Philosophical Fragments.* Edited and translated by Howard V. Hong and Edna H. Hong. Princeton, NJ: Princeton University Press, 1992.

———. *The Diary of Søren Kierkegaard.* Edited Peter P. Rohde. New York: Carol, 1993.

———. *The Point Of View, Etc.: Including The Point Of View For My Work As An Author, Two Notes About 'The Individual' And On My Work As An Author.* Translated by Walter Lowrie. New York: Oxford University Press, 1950.

———. *The Sickness Unto Death: A Christian Psychological Exposition For Upbuilding And Awakening.* Edited and translated by Howard V. Hong and Edna H. Hong. Princeton, NJ: Princeton University Press, 1980.

———. *Upbuilding Discourses in Various Spirits.* Edited and translated by Howard V. Hong and Edna H. Hong. Princeton, NJ: Princeton University Press, 1993.

———. *Works of Love.* Edited and Translated by Howard V. Hong and Edna H. Hong Princeton, NJ: Princeton University Press, 1995.

Pascal, Blaise. *Selections from the Thoughts, Pascal.* Edited and translated by Arthur H. Beattie. Arlington Heights, IL: Harlan Davidson, 1965.

Pirsig, Robert. *Zen and the Art of Motorcycle Maintenance: An Inquiry Into Values.* New York: HarperCollins, 2006.

Plato. *Parmenides and Theaetetus.* Translated by Benjamin Jowett. Washington, DC: Regnery, 1951.

———. *Phaedrus.* Indianapolis: The Library of Liberal Arts by Bobbs-Merrill, 1956.

———. *Symposium.* Translated by Alexander Nehamas and Paul Woodruff. Indianapolis: Hackett, 1989.

Roberts, Monty. *The Man Who Listens to Horses.* New York: Ballantine, 1997.

Shaw, Marvin. *The Paradox of Intention.* Atlanta: Scholars, 1988.

Thompson, Josiah. *Kierkegaard.* New York: Alfred A. Knopf, 1973.

Tzu, Lao. *Tao Te Ching.* Vintage Series. Translated by Gia-Fu Feng, Jane English, and Jacob Needleman. New York: Vintage, 1989.

Vlastos, Gregory. "Socratic Irony." *The Classical Quarterly,* New Series, 37 (1987) 79–96.

Walker, Alice. *Horses Make a Landscape Look More Beautiful.* Orlando: Harcourt Brace, 1979.

White, Elwyn Brooks, and Katharine Sergeant Angell White, eds. *A Subtreasury of American Humor.* New York: Pocket, 1941.

Wittgenstein, Ludwig. *Tractatus Logico-philosophicus.* Ann Arbor, MI: University of Michigan Press, 1922.

Yalom, Irving D., and Molly Leszcz. *The Theory and Practice of Group Psychotherapy.* New York: Basic, 2005.

www.ingramcontent.com/pod-product-compliance
Lightning Source LLC
Chambersburg PA
CBHW020830190426
43197CB00037B/1116